A RICH BIOETHICS

Notre Dame Studies in Medical Ethics

David Solomon, series editor

The purpose of the Notre Dame Studies in Medical Ethics series, sponsored by the Notre Dame Center for Ethics and Culture, is to publish works that specifically address contemporary issues in the field of medicine. The aim is to foster a systematic and rational discussion of medical ethical problems grounded in Catholic intellectual tradition and moral vision.

A RICH BIOETHICS

Public Policy, Biotechnology,

and the Kass Council

WITHDRAWN

ADAM BRIGGLE

University of Notre Dame Press

Notre Dame, Indiana

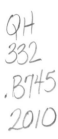

Manufactured in the United States of America

Library of Congress Cataloging-in-Publication Data

Briggle, Adam.
   A rich bioethics : public policy, biotechnology, and the Kass Council /
Adam Briggle.
      p.   cm. — (Notre Dame studies in medical ethics)
   Includes bibliographical references and index.
   ISBN-13: 978-0-268-02221-1 (pbk. : alk. paper)
   ISBN-10: 0-268-02221-6 (pbk. : alk. paper)
   1. Kass Council (U.S.)   2. Bioethics—Government policy—United States—
Case studies.   3. Bioethics—Philosophy.   4. Science and state—United States.
I. Title.
   QH332.B745   2010
   174'.9570973—dc22
                                                                    2010007654

∞ *The paper in this book meets the guidelines for permanence and durability*
of the Committee on Production Guidelines for Book Longevity of the Council
on Library Resources.

To Mary Grace:

with hope that you and your generation will

be wiser than your father and his.

Nature to be commanded must be obeyed.

—Francis Bacon, *Novum Organum*

Book I, Aphorism 3

CONTENTS

Acknowledgments   ix

Introduction: An Experiment in Public Bioethics   1

PART I   Rich Public Bioethics and the Kass Council

ONE   Public Bioethics and the Birth of the Kass Council   13

TWO   The Deeper History of the Kass Council   39

THREE   In Defense of Rich Public Bioethics I: Self and Society   61

FOUR   In Defense of Rich Public Bioethics II: Mind and Body   87

PART II   The Politics and Policy of Public Bioethics

FIVE   The Kass Council as Institution and Lightning Rod   115

SIX   The Politicization of Ethics Advice   131

SEVEN   The Kass Council as Humanities Policy   149

Conclusion: Public Philosophy in a Liberal Democracy   167

Notes   180

Works Cited   195

Index   214

ACKNOWLEDGMENTS

This work has evolved tremendously from its humble origins first as a seminar paper and then a Ph.D. thesis. Throughout this evolution I have benefited from the wise counsel, steadfast commitment, and good cheer of my colleagues, friends, and family. I was hesitant to pursue this project because American bioethics and science policy can be acrimonious affairs. I was afraid that I might be chewed up and spit out. Instead, I have had the good fortune to encounter only thoughtful, open-minded people in the course of my research. I believe this is because nearly everyone involved realizes the importance of these issues and wants above all to make a contribution to a serious and civil conversation about the ethics and politics of our world-transforming scientific knowledge and technological powers. I hope that this book will advance that conversation.

I wish to express my gratitude to everyone who has contributed to the profoundly educational experience of crafting this book. I am forever indebted to my friend and mentor Robert Frodeman, who diligently critiqued numerous versions of this text and provided insight and inspiration. His wisdom is matched only by the nobility of his soul, and often as we talked, dangling our feet in the clear and refreshing waters of Boulder Creek, I felt like the young Phaedrus with the great philosopher. Insofar as it succeeds in meeting the challenges of interdisciplinarity, this book is as much his as it is mine.

I am also deeply grateful for the friendship and professional mentoring of Carl Mitcham. It has been my distinct honor to work with him on this book and numerous other scholarly endeavors. It is rare to find someone so learned and so humble, so distinguished and so generous. I am further thankful for the sharp, pragmatic, and ever-challenging intelligence of Roger Pielke. His insights were particularly helpful in thinking through chapter 6, but I have tried to emulate his critical mindset throughout the text. James White and Lisa Keranen were also on my dissertation committee, and I am grateful for their comments and for encouraging me to pursue this topic further as a book.

I have worked on this book in two institutional homes. First, I benefited greatly from the resources at the Center for Science and Technology Policy Research at the University of Colorado, Boulder. In particular, I profited from countless conversations with fellow students including Shali Mohleji, Erik Fisher, Bets McNie, Genevieve Maricle, Jason Vogel, Nat Logar, Shep Ryen, Marilyn Averill, and Suzanne Tegen. Second, I have been supported by the Philosophy Department at the University of Twente, Enschede, the Netherlands. I am grateful to all of the members of this gadfly humanities department in a technological, entrepreneurial university. I would also like to thank Mark Brown, Summer Johnson, Gregor Wolbring, Robert Cook-Deegan, Steve Fuller, and Jennifer Brian, all of whom offered valuable feedback and stimulating discussions when I presented various portions of this book at conferences and workshops.

During my research, I attended some of the Kass Council meetings. I was pleased to find council members very approachable, and I am grateful for the opportunity to meet most of them. I am particularly thankful for the extended interviews granted by Leon Kass, Rebecca Dresser, Michael Gazzaniga, and Harold T. Shapiro, former chairman of NBAC. I found the council staff to be very helpful and professional, and I am especially indebted to Diane Gianelli for fielding my many queries and encouraging my efforts.

Finally, I would like to thank the reviewers for University of Notre Dame Press whose criticisms and recommendations improved this work enormously.

Introduction

An Experiment in Public Bioethics

Though his presidency would soon be dominated by the war on terrorism, in the summer of 2001 George W. Bush was focused on the war on disease. The U.S. and other developed countries have long committed national resources to biomedical research to improve the quality and extend the duration of human life. Although justified by an ethical commitment to well-being, federal support of biomedical science and technology raises ethical quandaries about how to distribute scarce resources and how to balance means and ends. By 2001 scientific advances and legislative activity in embryonic stem cell research had pushed such issues to the forefront of national consciousness and onto the president's agenda. Does the potential for cures justify the sacrifice of human embryos, the moral status of which is disputed in a pluralist society? Weighing on President Bush's mind was the more specific question of whether the federal government ought to fund embryonic stem cell research.

On August 9, 2001, in his first nationally televised address, President Bush announced his controversial decision. His policy would allow federal funding only on stem cell lines that existed prior to that day. Subsequent research developments have suggested that new techniques for creating stem cells may mitigate this moral controversy. But stem cells are only one aspect of a much larger constellation of ethical and political questions surrounding biomedical and behavioral science and technology. In recognition of this, President Bush took advantage of his national audience to announce the formation of the President's Council on Bioethics, which would "consider all of the medical and ethical ramifications of biomedical innovation." The council would be chaired by Dr. Leon Kass, a long-time contributor to and critic of bioethics.

"Bioethics" is a very recent coinage for discourse about very old questions concerning human identity, meaning, and flourishing—questions that are now raised with unprecedented urgency by modern biotechnology. These questions often provoke profoundly divergent answers that may in turn spark animosity. It may be that, in an ideal world, each person would be left alone to give his or her own private answers. But in the real world, substantive issues about being human cannot be banished from the public sphere. This is due in large part to the successes of modern science and technology. By drawing us into an ever more interdependent web and by delving into the very fabric of human nature, science and technology are forcing us to confront together questions about the nature of good lives and good societies. The central thesis of the present work is that since we cannot avoid such substantive matters, it is best to handle them explicitly. I will argue that this is what the Kass Council did and that this is what made it unique and important as an institution of public advice and public philosophy.

On November 28, 2001, President Bush signed executive order 13237, officially establishing the President's Council on Bioethics. The Kass Council finished its term on September 9, 2005, when Kass stepped down as its chairman.[1] Bioethics commissions are traditionally heavily influenced by their chairs, and the Kass Council was no exception. In terms of both substance and style, much of the council's work bears the unmistakable impress of Kass's thought. Indeed, Kass devoted himself nearly full-time to his council,[2] playing an integral role in the production of its seven official reports.

The council's mandate was broad: "to advise the President on bioethical issues that may emerge as a consequence of advances in biomedical science and technology," "to undertake fundamental inquiry into the human and moral significance of developments in biomedical and behavioral science and technology," "to provide a forum for a national discussion of bioethical issues," and "to facilitate a greater understanding of bioethical issues." As Kass put it at their first meeting in a Washington D.C. hotel on January 17, 2002, the council was to answer the demands for "action" in public policy and "thought" in public culture.[3] The council was thus tasked with fulfilling the needs for both policy-relevant information and philosophic reflection at the dawn of a new age of scientific discoveries and technological powers, from stem cell research and cloning to cognitive and physical enhancements.

Naturally the council would hold meetings, listen to testimony, and write reports just as previous bioethics committees had done. Such committees had existed in the U.S. since 1974, rising and falling with each change of presidential administration. But in his opening remarks at that first meeting, Kass made it clear that he wanted his council to break with this tradition of public bioethics as he perceived it. He envisioned a body that would practice a "richer and deeper public bioethics."[4] In membership, it was to be a council *on* bioethics, not *of* bioethicists. In method, it would consult literature and eschew the need for consensus in order to probe fundamental matters and offer a range of competing views. In substance, it would go beyond such specific issues as safety, justice, and informed consent in order to practice an overall philosophical anthropology, studying biomedicine within the context of the human lifeworld. These were the essential ingredients of Kass's experiment in public bioethics. The results were in many respects astonishing, especially considering the fact that most government advisory bodies live and die lodged in the bowels of bureaucracy. In contrast with this usual obscurity, printings of two of the council's reports, *Beyond Therapy* (Kass Council 2003a) and *Being Human* (Kass Council 2003b), could not keep up with demand, and the council became a lightning rod for political controversy.

Through an interdisciplinary case study of the Kass Council, this book aims to improve understanding of the relationships among philosophy, politics, science, and technology within democratic societies. Its primary audience is the bioethics community widely conceived, from those interested in philosophic issues to those concerned with the nuts and bolts of bioethical practice, especially as it takes shape in public bioethics institutions. The book will be of interest as well to those in science, technology, and society (STS) fields, particularly science and technology policy. Yet it is also aimed at the attentive public—those members of our society concerned with our common fate as we confront both the promises and the political and ethical dilemmas raised by science and technology.

The council is treated here as a *topos* or place interweaving perennial themes, contingent circumstances, and multiple perspectives. Comprising more than simply a case study, the topical approach explicitly recognizes the fluidity of social and epistemological categories, tracing the council's work across disciplinary boundaries and historical contexts. Understanding the Kass Council demands attentiveness to biomedical science and technology, the federal policy advisory system, the U.S. political and cultural landscapes, the historical development of bioethics as public advice and academic profession, and the philosophic underpinnings of the modern era with its emphasis on the production of scientific knowledge and the promotion of individual liberties. The Kass Council shows how these strands are increasingly interwoven. It set itself an interdisciplinary task within the context of a pluralist democracy facing profound decisions and disagreements about the meaning of human flourishing. The importance of the council lay in its unique perspective on how we ought to conceive and confront these decisions and disagreements—an instance of what I shall call "rich bioethics."

Outline and Argument

The purpose of this book is twofold, corresponding to its division into two parts. First and most importantly, it pictures the Kass Council as modeling a solution, rich bioethics, to a deeply rooted problem, and it defends the feasibility and importance of that solution. Second, the book pictures the Kass Council as a political institution of ethics advice within a polarized context and evaluates its performance in light of charges of inappropriate politicization and policy irrelevance. The conclusion offers a synthesizing story about the possible relationships between philosophers and a pluralist democratic society.

Comprising the first four chapters, part I argues that the Kass Council modeled a solution to a problem. The problem, in brief, is the way of thinking and talking about bioethics that I call "instrumentalism." As an approach to public bioethics, it is both undemocratic and inadequate. It is undemocratic because it excludes certain voices while privileging others without the benefit of open debate. Instrumentalism is inadequate because it offers a flattened conception of politics and what it means to be human, and trucks in a limited moral vocabulary incapable of evaluating the full import of the biomedical revolution. In short, instrumentalism is a poor framing of bioethics—it is a way of thinking and talking that is exclusionary and partial. Part I sets out a historical account of the emergence of the problem, diagnoses its shortcomings, and, using Kass Council reports, demonstrates the benefits of an alternative, richer framing of bioethics.

Chapter 1 surveys the history of U.S. public bioethics and the birth of the Kass Council, indicating how it both continued and sought to break with this tradition. Chapter 2 sets this proximal story in a deeper context. It identifies two modern myths at the core of instrumentalism. The first is that humans are pre-social beings, each equally rational and self-reliant. The second is that humans are reasoning minds unconnected to their affective bodies, or at least not connected in any morally significant way. But we are in fact interdependent and embodied creatures, and these facts about being human are proving to hold substantial ethical significance in the wake of biomedical progress. Thus, we require a richer public bioethics that can see clearly where the myths obscure. Chapters 3 and 4 demonstrate how the Kass Council's work developed this enhanced vision.

These myths also supply instrumental public bioethics with its two main theses. The first is about *public* bioethics—ethical inquiry supported by and housed within government—and holds that the only legitimate task for a bioethics commission is to treat matters of the right and to leave matters of the good to individual choice. The second is about *bioethics* and holds that a proceduralist moral language of risks, rights, and justice is sufficient for evaluating the ethical dimensions of biomedical science and technology. Individual rights, risks to physical well-being, and justice are important topics and will remain so. But they are not the whole story, and indeed where the myths misinform us about who we are, they stunt our understanding of what it means to be human, thereby distorting our ethical assessments of alternative choices. The burden of my defense of a rich *bioethics* is to show the need for a wider conceptual lens and a more robust ethical vocabulary to analyze biomedical science and technology. The burden of my defense of a rich *public* bioethics is to show that this kind of moral inquiry is an important and legitimate aspect of a liberal democratic government.

I set "rich bioethics" in contrast both to the "instrumentalist bioethics" practiced by previous commissions and a more general instrumentalist way of thinking prevalent in society. Instrumentalism is a mode of understanding with two essential aspects; it is "formal" and "isolationist." Rich ethical inquiry, by contrast, is "substantive" and "holistic."

As a formal mode of thinking, instrumentalism takes individual desires as private and uneducable and focuses on just procedures for adjudicating conflicts and ensuring the rights of individuals to safely seek the satisfaction of their given desires. It seeks the means to given ends. By contrast, the substantive nature of rich bioethics explicitly describes and evaluates ends, goods, or perspectives on the meaning of being human and living well. What matters, after all, is not just the freedom to choose, but choosing humanly worthy goals—choosing wisely and well. Rich bioethics therefore treats desires as amenable to education through the articulation and critique of assumptions about the good life. There are, then, *many* types of rich bioethics in terms of the substantive arguments put forward about human meaning and living well within the context of specific issues. The Kass Council considered several arguments that had been advanced by other thinkers and developed many of its own.

The holism of rich bioethics has three aspects, each of which expands on the isolationist approach. First, it treats the individual not as an atomistic subject engaged in social contracts, but as constituted by bonds of caring and obligation that shape identities and provide meaning to life. Second, it treats the human not as a disembodied will, but as a mixture of mind and body, reason and affection, both of which are ethically relevant to flourishing. Third, its focus is not on individual techniques or research programs considered in isolation, but rather on their human and social contexts and the cultural significance of science and technology writ large. In this manner, the holism of rich bioethics complements philosophy as argumentation with philosophy as raising awareness of ourselves and our situation. This is a task that philosophy shares with literature, as the council recognized in its own anthology of literature, *Being Human* (Kass Council 2003b).

The advantages of a rich approach to bioethics are that—in both its substantive inquiry and holistic outlook—it opens a more inclusive debate and extends critical thought beyond the artificial barriers erected by instrumentalism. It asks, for example, not just if it was a free and informed decision, but also whether it was a good decision. Or, as another example, it asks not just about the public policies called for by a technique, but also about its ramifications for culture, daily practice, identity, and character.

Yet a defense of rich public bioethics and some arguments made by the council is not a defense of the Kass Council as a political entity. As the idea of rich public bioethics takes institutional form, additional criteria are introduced—pertaining to procedures and conduct—by which to judge its appropriateness and success. Part II examines the Kass Council from this perspective, as a federal advisory body comprised of members and staff acting within political and historical contexts. Chapter 5 identifies important institutional features conducive to a rich public bioethics, surveys the political controversies surrounding the Kass Council, and introduces the major criticisms of politicization and irrelevance. Chapter 6 addresses the first criticism through three detailed case studies, concluding that charges of politicization were sometimes accurate, while at other times they were mischaracterizations. It is true that the council did not pay enough attention to its political context, procedures, and public image. But its detractors, in seeking to identify the work of the council as partisan politics by other means, largely refused to engage in substantive exchange with the council. Yet as part I argues, it is precisely this that the public and decision-makers most need in the face of complex ethical quandaries.

Chapter 7 investigates the charges of irrelevance by retrospectively making sense of the council's work as a form of "humanities policy." I use these charges as an opportunity to diagnose and critique an instrumentalist conception of public policy, thereby extending my analysis beyond bioethics to the broader arenas of science and technology policy. Policy instrumentalism is formal in seeing public policy in purely means-ends terms, and it is isolationist in conceiving of policy processes as discrete sequences of problems disembedded from culture and history. I argue that previous bioethics committees worked from within this image of policy, whereas the Kass Council implicitly critiqued its limitations. I use *Being Human* to demonstrate the policy relevance of the council's "rich humanities policy."

The Future of Public Bioethics

The greatest accomplishment of the Kass Council was its model of rich bioethics as a public forum and style of moral inquiry capable of both opening up and elevating debate. When implemented well, rich public bioethics promises to help citizens understand and contest the ethics and politics of biomedical science and technology. But the council did not perfectly institutionalize the idea of a rich public bioethics. It was widely perceived as politically co-opted and it did not do nearly enough to dispel this perception. Indeed, it sometimes reinforced this perception through inappropriate partisanship and faulty institutional design. Future commissions will need to be improved in several respects if they are to better implement the important idea of a rich public bioethics.

In June 2009, President Barack Obama ushered in the next phase of U.S. public bioethics by disbanding the President's Council on Bioethics. Predictably, the new Democratic White House framed its approach in stark contrast to the public bioethics of the preceding Republican administration. Most importantly, the Obama administration seemed to equate rich public bioethics with policy irrelevance. At the time, a White House spokesperson criticized the council for being "philosophically leaning" and failing to provide "practical policy options" (see Wade 2009). Five months later, in November 2009, Obama signed an executive order creating the Presidential Commission for the Study of Bioethical Isssues, to be chaired by Amy Gutmann. In announcing its formation, he stressed that it would develop "recommendations through practical and policy-related analyses." If the victors write history, then the Kass Council will be remembered as an arcane debating club that lost touch with the realities of public policy.

This judgment is a product of an instrumentalist mindset that sharply contrasts philosophic reflection and political action. But in an age of transformative biotechnology, policy decisions necessarily have philosophic dimensions about the meaning of being human and living well. How we think about ourselves and the moral language we bring to bear in our decisions are simultaneously philosophic and pragmatic issues. And at the risk of sounding faddish in a world that tends to "consume" everything, including its gurus and counselors, what we need most is the wisdom for living good lives in a hyperpaced world and the moral vision for governing burgeoning scientific and technological powers.

In short, far from losing touch with reality, the Kass Council cut to the heart of the questions posed by modern biotechnology: Who are we? Who do we wish to become and why? To dismiss these questions as navel-gazing is not to chase them from the public stage. Rather, it is to answer them in any given context surreptitiously with assumptions and prereflective preferences, oftentimes masked behind the veil of "objectivity." We must take care that, in seeking to be "practical," any future public bioethics is not simply swept along the margins of a technological and market imperative. We must take care that any future public bioethics remains a place to think together about the open question of the human condition, rather than a place where the answer is already presupposed.

PART I

Rich Public Bioethics
and the Kass Council

ONE

Public Bioethics
and the Birth of the Kass Council

In his 1784 essay "Answering the Question: What is Enlightenment?" Immanuel Kant articulated the spirit of the modern era: "Dare to know!" In this aphorism Kant expressed his conviction that deference to the natural order, authority, or received tradition hampers the maturation of humankind. Such servitude shows a lack of courage and a state of immaturity and dependence rather than the fortitude to use one's own intellect. Accordingly, Kant's moral philosophy emphasized autonomy, or the capacity of rational individuals to govern themselves independent of their places in a metaphysical or social order. For Kant, the individual rational will is the seat of an impulse to extend the frontiers of knowledge. It is the source of human dignity, and since it is shared by all human beings, it forms the basis for both freedom and justice and, thus, a modern liberal society.[1]

The daring that Kant spoke of has only one rational limitation. Knowledge may be allowed to transgress the dictates of authority, any belief in a natural order, and any interpretation of divine will. But individual pursuit of knowledge must not violate the autonomy of other persons. Enlightenment is about the pursuit of new knowledge, but this pursuit must respect individual rights, especially to physical well-being and social equality. If these conditions are satisfied, the currently popular reading of Kant holds that people can and should be able to do whatever they choose.

In the 1930s in Kant's homeland, the Nazi regime grew to power. According to Nazi ideology, the seat of human dignity lay not in the universally shared autonomous will, but in the physical characteristics of a certain race. Thus when the Nazi German physician Dr. Josef Mengele prowled the concentration camp at Auschwitz in the mid 1940s, he did not see autonomous individuals deserving of equal respect. Rather, the "Angel of Death," as the inmates called him, saw a lesser class of beings.

Mengele and other Nazi physicians performed atrocious experiments on concentration camp prisoners. The experiments included work on the effects of hypoxia, nerve gas, freezing, high pressure, and the ingestion of sea water. Prisoners were deliberately infected with bacteria in order to test untried compounds for medicinal qualities. Some physicians removed segments of bone, nerves, and other tissues and experimented with transplantations. Prisoners often died as a result of the experiments, or were murdered afterward and dissected. Many experiments were allegedly motivated by the desire to gain knowledge to improve the competitive edge of Nazi soldiers.

Following the war, international military courts put on trial twenty-three Nazi physicians in what came to be known as the twelve "Doctors' Trials," or the "Subsequent Nuremberg Trials."[2] In an appeal to a suprapositive principle transcending the laws of any one nation, the indictments referred to "crimes against humanity," which are grave affronts to human dignity. Prior to these trials, there were no statutes clearly distinguishing legal from illegal medical practices. Thus one of the key outcomes of the trials was the 1946 Nuremberg Code,[3] which sought to define legitimate medical research based on principles such as beneficence, which had long been a central aspect of medical ethics that could be traced back to the Hippocratic Oath of the fourth century BCE.

The Nuremberg Code, however, placed primary emphasis on the principle of informed consent, which had not been central to the Hippocratic tradition. Indeed, the first line of the Nuremberg Code reads: "The voluntary consent of the human subject is absolutely essential." This modern principle for the ethics of human experimentation is grounded in a

Kantian notion of autonomy—respect for the rights of rational individuals to be self-directed rather than determined by considerations imposed externally.[4] The Nuremberg Code led to the adoption of the Declaration of Geneva in 1948 by the World Medical Association (WMA). The WMA also adopted the Declaration of Helsinki in 1964, which outlined a set of ethical precepts and a guide to the protection of human rights in the conduct of experiments. These foundations of bioethics all shared a Kantian focus on autonomy and justice.

In addition to the ethics of human-subjects research, emerging biomedical technologies were impacting society in other, equally profound ways. Some notable examples include the era of genomics and molecular biology unleashed by the 1953 discovery of the double helical structure of DNA by Francis Crick and James Watson. The introduction of the birth control pill in 1960 and other assisted reproductive technologies (ART), including in vitro fertilization (IVF), wrought enormous societal changes. Biomedicine not only transformed the beginnings of human life, but its end as well, as the 1960s and 1970s witnessed "a dramatic shift from death at home to death in hospitals or other institutions" (Callahan 2004, 279). New technologies often gave physicians the power to produce effects that were not always beneficial for their patients. Doctors could now save lives that were compromised in some way, or be faced with the decision to save some lives at the expense of others. Thus the overriding question "to save or let die?" was first systematically treated by one of the founding figures in bioethics, James Childress, in his 1970 essay "Who Shall Live When Not All Can Live?" Advances in palliative care forced the question of when to withhold or withdraw life-sustaining treatments.

In the early 1960s, such questions were at the center of the renal dialysis debates. At that time, there were not enough machines to serve public demand and the issue, largely faced at the state level in the U.S., was how to distribute scarce resources. Some states used a lottery system, but in Seattle, Washington, a committee of citizens was formed to make these decisions.[5] Due to the gravity of the committee's deliberations, *Life* magazine dubbed it the "God Squad" (Alexander 1962). In a 1964 speech Dr. Belding Scribner, the inventor of renal dyalysis, predicted that the ethical problems his technique had encountered "will recur again and again as other new, complicated, expensive, life-saving techniques are developed."

In 1971 a short film made at Johns Hopkins University Hospital captured the agonizing decision to let an infant with Down's syndrome die, and sparked intense debate among physicians and ethicists.[6] In 1976 the case of Karen Ann Quinlan raised the ethics of life support and advance directives as well as the issue of how to define death (i.e., according to the cessation of cardiorespiratory, whole brain, or higher brain function). The Quinlan case was most famously discussed by theologian and ethicist Paul Ramsey (1976) in an essay entitled "Prolonged Dying: Not Medically Indicated." It raised the ethical dilemma concerning the difference between "letting die" and killing. The case was settled in the New Jersey Supreme Court, highlighting the fact that bioethical issues are often intertwined with the law. George Annas (1993) argues that this is because in a pluralist society there is no common set of beliefs or ethos about how to live rightly and well that could form the basis of any bio*ethics*.

The Prehistory of U.S. Public Bioethics

Although all of these society-science issues were occurring in the late 1960s and early 1970s, the creation of the first U.S. public bioethics commission was primarily sparked by an alarming array of controversial practices and outright scandals in research with human subjects. In 1974 the first U.S. bioethics commission was created and played a key role in formalizing, institutionalizing, and granting binding legal force to the kinds of principles outlined in the Nuremberg Code.[7]

Although the practices of the Nazi physicians were uniquely heinous, the unethical treatment of human subjects was not confined to the Nazi regime (see Rothman 2004). U.S. physicians also conducted questionable human experimentation during World War II, driven by the urgency to generate knowledge that could be of use to U.S. soldiers. Such practices continued throughout the 1960s and the early part of the 1970s, fuelled both by a continuing utilitarian outlook legitimated by the "war on disease" and by the increasingly impersonal relationship between the researcher and the patient as medicine grew into big business. A landmark whistle-blowing essay by anaesthesiologist and medical professor Henry Beecher in 1966, "Ethics and Clinical Research," identified over twenty unsettling practices and sparked a wider debate about the ethics of human experimentation. Beecher concluded that "unethical or questionably ethical procedures are not uncommon" among researchers.[8] German-American philosopher Hans Jonas (1969) contributed another defining essay in the ethics of medical research, which challenged the adequacy of utilitarian ethics. Academic philosophers thus were already preparing Kantian arguments from the inviolability of individuals to counter the overreaches of utilitarian projects that saw the exploitation of individuals as an acceptable means to social progress.

The Tuskegee Syphilis Experiment—exposed to the public in 1972— was perhaps the most dramatic of the scandals. Since 1932 the U.S. Public Health Service had conducted an experiment on 399 African American men in rural, impoverished Tuskegee, Alabama. (The hospital at the famous Tuskegee Institute was not a research partner, but did lend facilities and the services of at least one staff member, a nurse, on an occasional basis.) The patients were in the late stages of syphilis, and experiment was conducted without informed consent. In the latter part of the experiment, cheap and universally available treatments were withheld from the patients. As a result, the wives of some of the participants also contracted syphilis, and some of their children were born with congenital syphilis. But the Tuskegee Experiment was only one instance in a rash of unethical practices that culminated in public outrage and a legitimacy crisis for the medical research community. These included the Willowbrook Hepatitis Study (1963–1966), in which investigators fed live hepatitis viruses to the residents of an institution for the retarded in order to study the etiology of the disease and the possibilities of a vaccine. Another example involved physicians who, in 1963, injected live cancer cells into uninformed elderly and senile patients at the Brooklyn Jewish Chronic Disease Hospital in order to study the body's immunological responses. Another case was the 1967 "Tea Room Trade," which violated the privacy of subjects in a study of homosexual subcultures.[9]

As the number and severity of these abuses of power became widely known, a political atmosphere developed in which self-regulation by biomedical scientists and the medical profession was increasingly questionable. The professional codes of medical ethics were insufficient to address larger policy and ethical issues.[10] The later Quinlan case only confirmed for many in the public a sense that patients did not understand what the era of high-tech medicine meant for them. This apprehension took the shape of a general concern that patient autonomy was not being respected (Jecker 1997). It was becoming apparent that greater oversight and awareness were necessary to direct the burgeoning revolution in medicine.

Throughout many of the scandals, the government had played a passive and ad hoc role. But in 1966, the U.S. National Institutes of Health (NIH) created a decentralized system of regulations that for the first time established collective surveillance over decisions traditionally delegated to individual physicians. At the core of this system were review committees known as institutional review boards (IRBs)—decentralized group boards composed partially of nonscientists that review the ethics of research proposals involving human subjects. The U.S. Food and Drug Administration (FDA) went further in distinguishing between therapeutic and nontherapeutic research. The FDA prohibited the latter unless patients gave consent, a concept that the FDA explicitly elaborated to a greater extent than the NIH.

Yet the research scandals had broader implications than increased regulations. As theologian Paul Ramsey argues, society can no longer "go on assuming that what can be done has to be done or should be. . . . These questions are now completely in the public forum, no longer the province of scientific experts alone" (Ramsey 1970, 1). Ethical questions surrounding medicine and biomedical research could no longer be sheltered from public debate. The notion of "consent" was broadened beyond the individual patient-physician relation to include informed social consent to the pace, scale, and direction of biomedical research that was turning society at large into a laboratory. Pressure was building for improved accountability, policy guidance, and wider discussion. Public bioethics commissions emerged as one possible response to this pressure.

John Fletcher and Franklin Miller argued that such committees essentially serve two functions: "promotion of accountability and enlarging foresight amidst bioethical controversies" (Fletcher and Miller 1996, 174). First, commissions could serve as "a forum for developing ethical standards to assure public accountability in biomedical research, healthcare, and public health" (Fletcher and Miller 1996, 156). A publicly mandated commission with diverse representation would be "an appropriate vehicle for recommending guidelines for reviewing, monitoring, and conducting research to be incorporated into government regulations" (Fletcher and Miller 1996, 156). Bioethics commissions could help to ensure the integrity and accountability of scientific research and to negotiate claims to authority and legitimacy in matters of science policy, roles increasingly played by organizations at the boundaries of science and politics (see Guston 2000; Kelly 2003).

Second, in addition to advising the regulation of present research, bioethics commissions can be thought of as proactively contemplating the ethics of future research. They could "serve the need of government for intelligence and counsel on emerging ethical problems, spawned by advances in scientific knowledge and technology" (Fletcher and Miller 1996, 156). In technological societies, citizens expect policymakers to consult experts to enhance the quality and credibility of decision making. This has led to the formation of federal advisory bodies, which have been collectively termed "the fifth branch" of government (see Jasanoff 1990). Such bodies were almost exclusively technical in nature until the formation of bioethics commissions, which by their very name and purposes broadened the fifth branch to include philosophic, ethical, and theological expertise. General, federal-level bioethics committees have traditionally had no regulatory authority.[11] They narrow, expand, articulate, or assess different ethical positions and policy options. They are not charged with deciding right and wrong (i.e., making policy).[12]

Yet as the federal government began to contemplate its need for greater counsel and foresight, another kind of Kantian concern arose: fears within the scientific community about a loss of professional autonomy. Policy makers found it difficult to garner support among scientists and physicians for the idea of a public bioethics commission. Albert Jonsen (1998), a member of the first bioethics commission and a Jesuit priest at that time, traced this conflict back to a series of hearings conducted in 1968 by the Subcommittee on Government Research of the Senate Committee on Government Operations. They were initiated by Senator Walter Mondale (D-MN), who cited genetic engineering and heart transplantation[13] as specific areas that pointed to a need for a national discussion on the direction of medical science. Mondale proposed a commission to study a broad range of medical advances that "raise grave and fundamental ethical and legal questions for our society. Who shall live and who shall die?

How long shall life be preserved and how should it be altered? Who will make decisions? How shall society be prepared?" (in Jonsen 1998, 91).

The testimony of the scientists that appeared before the committees provides a telling look into society-science relations, as scientists maneuvered to define and defend their jurisdiction. Some scientists liked the idea of a commission because it might allay public fears, thus playing a legitimizing (but not a deeply scrutinizing) role for the further advancement of biomedical research. But almost all were reluctant to concede that medical advances presented any serious ethical problems, at least not in the near term, and many argued that the scientific community could police itself. The prevalence of this stance prompted Mondale at one point to retort in exasperation that biochemist Arthur Kornberg seemed reluctant "to have persons other than the people in your laboratory look at the social implications" (in Jonsen 1998, 91). Taking a minority stance among the scientific community, Nobel laureate biologist Joshua Lederberg enthusiastically pictured a commission that would "foster a continuing debate," thus keeping matters of ultimate value open to reflection and discussion. Theologians who testified also sought to define and expand their jurisdiction by proposing a commission that would take a radical look at the stakes of the technological conquest of human nature.

Many scientists were openly hostile to Mondale's proposal. The surgeon Christiaan Barnard, who performed the first heart transplant surgery, spoke most candidly about how such a commission, if it were anything more than a group of scientists and doctors, would set U.S. science far behind international competition. In response to a Senator's concern that the public was paying for much of the research and deserved a voice, Dr. Barnard replied, "Who pays the cost of war? The public! Who decides where the general should attack? The public? The public is not qualified to make the decision. The general makes the decision. He is qualified to spend the public's money the best way he thinks fit" (in Jonsen 1998, 92). For Barnard, only medical doctors and scientists qualify as "the general," certainly not representatives of the public or of any other type of expertise (e.g., ethical or theological). Owen Wangensteen, a professor of surgery, similarly expressed concern that a commission would unnecessarily shackle scientific freedoms. When asked if nonphysicians had any valuable input, he replied, "the fellow who holds the apple can peel it best" (in Jonsen 1998, 93).

The Mondale hearings did little more than simply "air" the issues, and no bioethics commission resulted. But in a stunning subsequent development, 1973 NIH recommendations[14] encouraged the use of live fetuses for medical research before they died. This move sparked public protests and a further round of hearings in the Senate Committee on Labor and Public Welfare chaired by Senator Edward Kennedy (D-MA), as well as by other congressional committees. Foreshadowing the major role that bioethics would come to play in American politics, these hearings garnered nearly unprecedented levels of media coverage. Referring to neurological, pharmacological, and genetic research, Senator Kennedy began the first hearing by declaring that "scientists may stand on the threshold of being able to recreate man" (in Fox and Swazey 2008, 49). He reconfirmed Congressional commitment to broader oversight, claiming that policy must be shaped not just by medical professionals, but also by ethicists, theologians, and others.

The idea of a commission again became a large part of these deliberations, partially for the reasons noted above and partially as a way for political leaders to take symbolic action and skirt difficult decisions that fringed the abortion debate. Given the growing presence of advisory bodies in government and the increasing controversies about biomedical research, the idea of an advisory commission began to build widespread support among politicians, the general public, and many ethicists and theologians.

The Rise of U.S. Public Bioethics: The National Commission and Principlism

On July 12, 1974, drawing from the Kennedy hearings, Congress passed the National Research Act, which prohibited federal funding for any research that violated NIH standards, and included an amendment prohibiting research on any fetus with "a beating heart." Part of this public law mandated the creation of the temporary National Commission for the Protection of Human Subjects of Biomedical and Behavioral Research (National Commission), chaired by Kenneth J. Ryan, M.D. Congress charged it with identifying "basic ethical principles" to guide biomedical research involving human subjects, including the articulation of the theoretical principles upon which previous regulations were based.

The National Commission was composed of eleven members drawn from both "the general public" and experts from scientific and nonscientific disciplines including philosophy, law, and theology. No more than five of the members could be researchers, again indicating Congressional commitment to bring human experimentation under outside scrutiny. The National Commission was primarily mandated to cover issues of human-subject research. It produced reports on research involving vulnerable subjects including prisoners, those institutionalized as mentally infirm, fetuses, and children. It was the first federal-level U.S. public bioethics institution,[15] its task formally defined as "ethical inquiry conducted by a publicly constituted body, which is created and supported by government" (Fletcher and Miller 1996, 155).

Administered by the NIH within the Department of Health, Education, and Welfare (DHEW), the National Commission operated until 1978. Though it had no enforcement powers of its own, it advised on the first federal regulations for the protection of human subjects of biomedical and behavioral research (45CFR46).[16] In 1979, the DHEW adopted these regulations, known as the Belmont Report (National Commission 1979), as a statement of its policy regarding the ethics of research involving human subjects. The regulations and principles outlined in the Belmont Report are principally institutionalized in the IRBs.[17]

The three principles described by the Belmont Report are: "respect for persons," "justice," and "beneficence." The principle of "respect for persons" is defined as "the requirement to acknowledge autonomy and the requirement to protect those with diminished autonomy." The principle of "beneficence" is an obligation to secure a patient's well-being, or "(1) do not harm and (2) maximize possible benefits and minimize possible harms." The principle of justice pertains primarily to fairness in distributing the burdens and benefits of medical research. The Belmont Report gave rise to a predominant form of bioethics known as "principlism."

As Jonsen wrote, the Belmont Report "had a major impact on the development of bioethics. Its principles found their way into the general literature of the field, and, in the process grew from the principles underlying the conduct of research into the basic principles of bioethics" (Jonsen 1998, 104).[18] The principle of "respect for persons" has since become an important and contested centerpiece of bioethics. Within clinical and academic bioethics, it has been reduced in many respects to a principle of respect for "autonomy," especially after the 1979 publication of Tom Beauchamp and James Childress's hugely influential textbook, *Principles of Biomedical Ethics.* Through this work, principlism became a leading approach in academic bioethics, but many other approaches—including those inspired by feminism, communitarianism, and various theological and conservative traditions—also grew alongside it and often competed with one another in professional journals (see e.g., Clement 1996; Callahan 2003; Breck and Breck 2005).

By contrast, until the Kass Council, public bioethics committees largely examined issues—often extending beyond the scope of human-subjects research—from within a mostly principlist framework. This was due in part to the argument that the task of such bodies is to forge consensus and offer advice on practical issues, which is well facilitated by these abstract principles (see Ainslie 2004; Brock 2004). Beauchamp and Childress were both working with the National Commission as they were drafting their book. They argued that agreement could be found at the level of principles even when disagreement persisted at the higher level of theory.

Principlism has since matured to take into account formal criticisms (e.g., Jonsen and Toulmin 1988; Clouser and Bernard 1990). Most importantly, later editions of *Principles of Biomedical Ethics* acknowledge the importance of casuistic reasoning in specific cases and reflective equilibrium in situations where the principles clash or are unclear (Davis 1995). This is particularly important with regard to the principle of respect for persons, which, as the Belmont Report notes, goes beyond autonomy: "The capacity for self-determination matures during an individual's life, and some individuals lose this capacity wholly or in part because of illness, mental disability, or circumstances that severely restrict liberty." The report goes on to note that "respect for the immature and the incapacitated may require protecting them as they mature or while they are incapacitated."

Thus, it is not sufficient to replace respect for *persons* with respect for *autonomy,* because in many situations patients or research subjects are not fully autonomous and *respect* may call for judicious protection rather than just informed consent. Indeed, the history of research ethics is laden with protectionism. For example, the bioethics commission established by President Bill Clinton (see below) recommended prohibiting experiments on human reproductive cloning in order to protect "the fetus and/or potential child"—notwithstanding the possibility of obtaining informed consent from the cell donors or from the prospective parents of a child created via cloning. This is a clear case where the principle of beneficence conflicts with an autonomy-oriented interpretation of respect for persons. Practitioners confront the difficulties in "applying" this principle in other areas, as well. This is the case, for example, with the recent growth in "guinea pigging," the practice of healthy people earning a living by volunteering for drug-safety trials (Elliott 2008).

One way to put the matter is that there are thin and thick notions of autonomy. Stephen Pinker (2008) articulates the thin notion, where autonomy "amounts to treating people in the way that they wish to be treated." This is an attempt to make the principle of respect for persons as simple as gathering informed consent. But from its beginnings in the Belmont Report, public bioethics could not rest satisfied with this thin notion. The hard cases presented by coercion, incapacity, illness, or immaturity raise the need to reflect on a thick, or rich, notion of autonomy. Indeed, quite the opposite of Pinker, Kant argues that humans act heteronomously if they act on the basis of the desires that they happen to have rather than in accordance with their rational wills. As the Belmont Report notes, for example, prisoners may be subtly coerced—perhaps without them even realizing it—into "volunteering" for drug-safety trials. In this way, principlism necessitates fundamental thinking about the principles themselves: What are respect, personhood, and autonomy? What does it mean in a given situation to act respectfully? This is important in looking ahead to the Kass Council, because, seen from this perspective, it did not so much break with the tradition of principlism in public bioethics as continue to delve deeper into the kind of richer thinking that it invites.

The Eclipse and Renewal of Public Bioethics

One of the recommendations of the National Commission led to the creation in 1978 of the second bioethics commission, the Ethics Advisory Board (EAB), chaired by James Gaither, J.D., and operating within the DHEW. During its approximately two-year existence, the EAB focused on issues involving fetuses, pregnant women, and in vitro fertilization (IVF), but it also had a broad charter that allowed it to investigate many bioethical topics. Originally intended as an ongoing, standing board, the EAB was nonetheless disbanded in 1980 after producing four documents. Two major outcomes were the stipulation of criteria for federally funded IVF research[19] (thus affirming that basic human embryo research including laboratory development of embryos was ethically acceptable under certain circumstances) and a pronouncement on human embryo research. The EAB traveled the country, holding public hearings and inviting citizens to testify on these matters. The termination of the EAB created a de facto ban on federal funding for human embryo research (which lasted for roughly fifteen years), as all such proposals had to be reviewed by the now nonexistent EAB.

One of the reasons for disbanding the EAB was that policy makers could not distinguish its purposes from those of the third committee, the President's Commission for the Study of Ethical Problems in Medicine and Biomedical and Behavioral Research (President's Commission) created in 1978 by Congress under Democratic president Jimmy Carter (see Gray 1995). The President's Commission, chaired by Morris B. Abram, J.D.,[20] produced ten reports over four years. It had a broader mission than the National Commission and the authority to initiate its own reports on emerging issues judged important by its members. It was elevated to independent presidential status. Also unlike the previous committees, the President's Commission produced fewer specific recommendations targeted at federal agencies. Instead, it produced consensus reports based on perceptions of the mainstream views of U.S. citizens.

These reports were and remain highly regarded, and "many have had sustained policy influence" (USOTA 1993, 12). Its reports *Defining Death* (President's Commission 1981) and *Deciding to Forgo Life-sustaining Treatment* (President's Commission 1983) were the most influential, and they strengthened the case for living wills, which again highlights the central role played by the principle of respect for autonomy. This is also apparent in its report *Making Health Care Decisions* (1982), which is entirely devoted to the principle of informed consent. *Securing Access to Health Care* (1983) emphasizes the principle of justice. After a three-month extension, the President's Commission expired in March 1983 under Republican president Ronald Reagan.

The Biomedical Ethics Advisory Committee (BEAC) was the fourth government-sponsored general bioethics body. In 1986 Congress established the Biomedical Ethics Board (BEB), which was composed of six Senators and six Representatives.[21] It took the BEB more than two years to appoint all the members of the BEAC, and in September 1988 (less than a week before it was originally scheduled to expire) the BEAC held its first meeting. Due largely to the politics of abortion, the appropriations for the BEAC were frozen and it was unable to produce any reports before it officially expired in September 1989 under Republican president George H. W. Bush. It held only two meetings, thus highlighting the politically contentious nature of such commissions, the difficulty of using them to address deeply divisive issues, their vulnerability to partisan politicization, and the diversity of ways for drafting their missions and selecting members.

The stillborn BEAC initiated an extended period without a general public bioethics commission. Fletcher and Miller argued that this "eclipse of public bioethics" was harmful for several reasons. Most importantly, they contended, "Power used to intervene in bioethical controversies, without being informed by the process of public bioethics, is bound to be perceived by many as abusive. Investigators and clinicians with vested interests in the activities involved will be more willing to accept regulatory limitations if these are the consequence of a process of public deliberation" (Fletcher and Miller 1996, 164).

Fletcher and Miller claimed that the Reagan and first Bush administrations tended to create policies on biomedical research and healthcare based on moral opposition to certain actions without open public debate. They made an important ethical claim that in the morally divisive and confusing contexts of biomedical science and technology policy, higher-quality decision-making outcomes and processes result from principled arguments "constrained by norms of informed debate, shared decision making, and enlarging foresight that flourished in public bioethics in an earlier period" (Fletcher and Miller 1996, 166). Indeed, improving the democratic forums of deliberation and decision making through such activities is the central goal of federal bioethics commissions.

To call this period an "eclipse" of public bioethics, however, is a misnomer. This was actually a time of rich debate about the purposes and mechanisms of public bioethics. It was during this period that the U.S.

Office of Technology Assessment produced the most comprehensive over-view of U.S. public bioethics (USOTA 1993). Such self-conscious scrutiny tends to subside as bioethics commissions become a routine part of government. More importantly, ad hoc, topic-specific advisory committees and decentralized local oversight and regulatory committees such as IRBs, hospital ethics committees (HECs), and the Recombinant DNA Advisory Committee (RAC) continued to fulfill oversight and monitoring functions. New York and New Jersey also established state-level bioethics committees.

Though centralized blue-ribbon national committees were in an eclipse, this decentralized network flourished. Bioethics committees and ethics councils in other nations also multiplied, inspired by the success of the U.K. Warnock Committee (1982–1984) on assisted reproduction (see Poland 1998; Fuchs 2005; UNESCO 2005; Ahvenharju et al. 2006). Moreover, the 1980s and early 1990s witnessed the growth of alternative practices for anticipating and discussing the ethical and social dimensions of science and technology. This included the establishment in 1988 of the Ethical, Legal, and Societal Impacts (ELSI) program chaired by Nancy Wexler. The ELSI program was part of the U.S. federal Human Genome Project (HGP). As the principal agencies involved in the HGP, the Department of Energy (DOE) and the NIH devoted between three and five percent of the HGP budgets to the study of social, legal, and ethical issues (see Juengst 1996). This created the world's largest bioethics program up to that time. It included an advisory committee that was subjected to charges of politicization in ways that recalled the troubles of the BEAC and foreshadowed those of the Kass Council.

During this time a debate also ensued about the need for a central-ized commission. The debate played out most succinctly in 1994 in the pages of the journal *Politics and the Life Sciences*. Some (e.g., Blank 1994) argued against a centralized bioethics committee on the ground that a de-centralized system could provide a broader airing of policy ideas without sacrificing the ability to provide authoritative guidance. Others (e.g., Carmen 1994) rejected the idea of a national bioethics panel because it threatened to remove policymaking power from elected representatives and was too far removed from the concrete contexts in which ethical inquiry could gain traction. Thus, for some, a distributed system of oversight bodies attached to specific research proposals and specific contexts made the most sense. Some argued that the OTA (now defunct), the National Academy of Science (NAS), or academic ethics institutions such as the Hastings Center could serve the same role as a national bioethics commission (e.g., Blank 1994; Cohen 1994).

Deborah Mathieu flatly stated her "doubt that any national bioethics panel would be sufficiently helpful or authoritative to justify the time, expense, and effort required" (Mathieu 1994, 91). To be successful, a commission designed to incorporate ethics into policymaking must be widely perceived as legitimate, but "in our pluralistic and deeply divided society, would we really trust these elites to make such delicate, value-laden decisions for us?" (Mathieu 1994, 91). This issue of elite "philosopher kings" or "wise man councils" defining ethical matters in a pluralistic society has been an enduring element of debates surrounding public bioethics (e.g., Dzur and Levin 2004; Evans 2006). The reply of those who support bioethics commissions has been that they must be independent and composed of diverse, dispassionate members in order to secure legitimacy in the eyes of the public.

Mathieu pointed out an apparent catch-22 in the arguments of those supporting national bioethics commissions. Some argued that such panels could only successfully resolve relatively noncontentious issues. For example, Cynthia Cohen (1994) argued that a federal commission is unlikely to develop recommendations and receive public support unless "sufficient consensus had developed." But Mathieu retorted that "if the issues are so straightforward, must we go to the expense of supporting a commission and its professional staff to resolve them?" (Mathieu 1994, 91). She further questioned how authoritative commissions can be if, as has happened,[22] their reports sometimes contradict one another. National bioethics commissions may produce the same incoherent patchwork of guidelines yielded by the more distributed system of institutions, especially as they tend to rise and fall with presidents and their political parties. Others later argued that ethics committees focus too much on outcomes and not enough on the democratic deliberative process of working through complex issues (Brown 2006).

Yet many maintained there was a need to resurrect a centralized bioethics commission. The strongest argument from this camp was put forth by three researchers who had collaborated on the OTA report (Hanna,

Cook-Deegan, and Nishimi 1993; 1994). In a response to some of the above critiques, they argued that members of both political parties recognized a need for a national commission, which signaled a politically palpable policy vacuum. The National Commission, they argued, had provided a model forum for moving from abstract principles to more specific guidelines upon which regulations could be based. The hugely influential Belmont Report provided the best example of how ethics experts could translate complex philosophical and religious issues into effective federal regulations (USOTA 1993; Fletcher and Miller 1996; Jonsen 1998). The three authors also argued that national bioethics commissions provide much-needed "broad-ranging and public discussion" that could "enrich and discipline the democratic debate." Moreover, "an authoritative and credible commission would act as a counterbalance to interest group and partisan politics" (Hanna, Cook-Deegan, and Nishimi 1994, 105). A national commission could command the authority and resources needed to address issues that required expansive access to information and expertise (USOTA 1993).[23] Others in the bioethics community also proposed resurrecting the national commission model of public bioethics (e.g., Fletcher 1994; Gray 1995). This debate worked to highlight the array of different roles to be served by bioethics commissions and the different standards to evaluate their success.

The dispute about the value of national bioethics commissions took on a new dimension in 1995 when President Bill Clinton signed an executive order to create the fifth bioethics committee, the National Bioethics Advisory Commission (NBAC). This decision arose in part out of recommendations made by the Advisory Committee on Human Radiation Experiments (1994–1995), which was a hybrid bioethics commission and "truth commission" with the authority to investigate the role of the U.S. government in human radiation experiments.[24] The proponents of a national bioethics committee won the debate in part because of the ability of such an institution to provide advice and to facilitate an enriched public understanding of bioethical issues. But these committees were also politically expedient. Creating a commission is in some measure a symbolic act signaling that political leaders have identified a problem, even if no further policy action is taken as a result of the committee's deliberations. Furthermore, political leaders can use such commissions to legitimate foregone conclusions with the patina of open debate or to stall on morally divisive issues by shifting their treatment, at least temporarily, into the hands of experts.

Clinton's NBAC executive order required that three out of the eighteen committee members be selected from the "general public." Chaired by Harold T. Shapiro, president of Princeton University and a professor of economics and public health policy, NBAC held its first meeting in 1996, and its original mission was to investigate two priority areas—human-subjects research and genetic information. Following the cloning of the sheep Dolly in 1996, however, President Clinton requested a report on cloning.[25] Dolly embodied one of the most important justifications for public bioethics: our technological powers often arrive far ahead of our ability to understand their implications, creating a need to cope with the resulting "future shock" (Toffler 1970).

The cloning report, the first of seven reports produced by NBAC, recommended that federal regulations be enacted to ban research using cloning, technically known as somatic cell nuclear transfer (SCNT), to create children (NBAC 1997). Importantly, the justification for this ban was that cloning techniques were unsafe. Thus it was based on a certain weighting of the Belmont principles of beneficence and autonomy. NBAC also recommended that such legislation be crafted so as not to interfere with other uses of cloning that might not be as ethically problematic. In its *Ethical and Policy Issues in Research Involving Human Participants* (2001), NBAC further emphasized the principles of beneficence (weighing risks and benefits) and autonomy (informed consent). The NBAC report on stem cells (1999) recommended that federal funding be used for research on stem cells derived from only two sources: cadaveric fetal tissue and embryos remaining after infertility treatments. NBAC expired in 2001 with the end of the Clinton administration.

The Kass Council

On November 28, 2001, President George W. Bush signed executive order 13237, establishing the President's Council on Bioethics as the sixth general federal bioethics commission. While the president's order actuated the council, developments in the preceding years had been formative to its concerns.

In 1993 Congress enacted the NIH Revitalization Act, which opened the way in principle to the possibility of NIH funding for human embryo research using IVF embryos. This Act rescinded the requirement that research protocols be approved by the disbanded EAB. The NIH Human Embryo Research Panel recommended federal funding for: (a) some forms of human embryo research on IVF embryos, and (b) the creation of human embryos for research purposes only. President Clinton overruled the latter recommendation, but accepted the former.

Congress, however, did not endorse either policy, and in 1996 created a provision that came to be known as the "Dickey Amendment," which prohibited the use of federal funds for research that destroys or seriously endangers human embryos or creates them for research purposes. Because it was attached to an appropriations bill, the Dickey Amendment required annual renewal.[26] In 1998 scientists at the University of Wisconsin[27] derived embryonic stem cells for the first time, which increased pressure for federal investment in this potentially promising line of medical research. In 1999 the General Counsel of the Department of Health and Human Services suggested that the Dickey Amendment could be interpreted to allow federal funding of stem cell research as long as the embryos were not destroyed using federal funds. The Clinton administration adopted this interpretation but did not have time to implement it before the end of its second term. Many conservatives remained concerned that this policy violated the spirit of the law. In a related development, in 2001 the U.S. House of Representatives passed a strict ban on all human cloning, including the production of cloned human embryos that could act as another source of stem cells.[28]

Upon entering office in January 2001, President Bush prioritized the closely related developments of cloning and embryonic stem cell research by putting the new regulations (developed by the Clinton administration but never implemented) on hold, pending a review. In July 2001, the president met with several people engaged in bioethics debates. These included Leon Kass, who was then professor at the University of Chicago and who had served as a fellow at the American Enterprise Institute for Public Policy Research, and Daniel Callahan, who was the head of the Hastings Center on Bioethics. The philosopher Larry Arnhart argued that because "Kass expressed . . . skepticism about modern science and technology in his published writings, he won the respect of American political and religious conservatives who shared his suspicion that the modern scientific project was subverting the moral and religious traditions inherited from antiquity" (Arnhart 2005, 1483). The drafting of the executive order and the formation of the council were nontransparent, but it would appear that this meeting and consonance of beliefs led to Kass's appointment as chair of the council.

On August 2, 2001, NIH officials made the now controversial report to President Bush that the number of existing stem cell lines was more than twice as great as previously believed. On August 9, in his first nationally televised address, the president announced his stem cell decision[29] in conjunction with his plan to form the council. In the address he stated: "As the discoveries of modern science create tremendous hope, they also lay vast ethical mine fields. As the genius of science extends the horizons of what we can do, we increasingly confront complex questions about what we should do. We have arrived at that brave new world that seemed so distant in 1932, when Aldous Huxley wrote about human beings created in test tubes in what he called a 'hatchery.'"

After announcing his stem cell decision, President Bush continued:

> I will also name a president's council to monitor stem cell research, to recommend appropriate guidelines and regulations, and to consider all of the medical and ethical ramifications of biomedical innovation. This council will consist of leading scientists, doctors, ethicists, lawyers, theologians and others, and will be chaired by Dr. Leon Kass. This council will keep us apprised of new developments and give our nation a forum to continue to discuss and evaluate these important issues. As we go forward, I hope we will always be guided by both intellect and heart, by both our capabilities and our conscience.

In November 2001 researchers at Advanced Cell Technologies in Massachusetts reported that they had created the first human embryo clones. At that point, according to one report, "the paperwork flew" to form the council (Weiss 2002). President Bush signed the executive order later that month and announced the members of the council on the night of January 16, 2002. This was the first time the names had been made public. The council members held their first meeting the next morning.

The nontransparent nature of the council's prehistory (i.e., chair, membership, and mission selection) immediately raised suspicions of bias. The council staff suggested that the level of transparency was typical of the formation of bioethics commissions by previous presidents.[30] Though true, this explanation does not address why and how the members were chosen or why a general ethics commission was formed rather than a more topic-specific initiative on stem cell research and cloning. Kass (2005) would later regret the heavy influence of stem cells and cloning at the genesis of the council, because he felt it skewed perceptions of the council's role (as stated in the executive order) of conducting ethical inquiry about a much broader range of topics.

Instrumental and Rich Public Bioethics

The history of U.S. public bioethics is complex and nuanced. Commissions each worked within their own context and had different memberships, missions, and institutional characteristics. In this sense, each commission was "an experiment in public bioethics." Nonetheless, there is one major theme running throughout the story. It is a theme that might have been lost in the noise had it not been for the thorough content analysis of John Evans (2002) in his description of "the rationalization of public bioethical debate" over the last quarter of the twentieth century.[31]

Evans's thesis is that public bioethics commissions and the professional bioethicists who increasingly shaped their work contributed to a "thinning" of the public bioethical debate. By this, he means that a "substantively rational" discourse about bioethical issues was displaced by a "formally rational" discourse. Substantive rationality asks whether the means are consistent with ultimate ends or values: "ends and means are debated as a piece" (Evans 2002, 13). By contrast, formal rationality asks whether the means employed are being maximized to achieve assumed ends. Partly as a result of the rise of public and professional bioethics, a discussion about ends and goods was largely displaced by a discussion about the means to ensure the assumed ends of autonomy, beneficence, and justice. In the 1960s and early 1970s, prior to the first bioethics commissions, a substantive public debate was predominant. For example, geneticist Theodosius Dobzhansky and other scientists spoke of "taking control of human evolution," a move that theologian Paul Ramsey called a sign of dangerous "messianic positivism."[32] After the rise of professional and public bioethics, however, formal rationality dominated bioethical discourse.[33] As it is a means-ends form of inquiry, I shall call the product of this thinning "instrumentalism."

Explaining why instrumentalism is problematic—and thus why the Kass Council was an important corrective—gets to the heart of what public bioethics does and what it should be. As noted above, the role of public bioethics institutions has long been debated (e.g., Dzur and Levin 2007; Johnson 2007). I will here briefly offer my own formulation of the proper role of public bioethics. Chapters 3 and 4 will further illustrate and defend the claims made here.

Public bioethics institutions hold meetings and produce reports that are available for the general public. Even if the primary intended audience is policy makers, the recommendations are widely available. Thus public bioethics institutions shape the structure of the debate and the views of the public that they claim to represent. Whether offering targeted advice or a broader discussion, bioethics committees model a way of thinking and talking about bioethical matters, or a way of framing complex questions and conflicting views. In this way they influence the quality of public understanding and discussion.

The thinning of public bioethics imposes strict limitations on public debate: only certain ends are considered a legitimate part of the discursive frame. This limitation has been justified by appeals to pluralism (see Engelhardt 1996; Ainslie 2004). American society is composed of many, often conflicting, visions of the good life. In order to accommodate these differences, public and professional bioethics created a "neutral" moral language (primarily of risks and rights) rather than justify proposed solutions to moral problems through appeal to a particular moral tradition or to complex philosophical theories. Each community can use a thicker moral language of the good internally, but then must translate this into the "common morality" or "overlapping consensus" developed within public bioethics when attempting to justify policies that affect all Americans. According to this view, then, the thinning of public bioethics protects democratic pluralism.

But the thinning of public bioethical debate is in fact antithetical to democratic pluralism, which is better served by a rich public bioethics. As Evans notes, the limitation on discourse has not been neutral. Rather, it has favored the interests of some groups over others, allowing some forms of discourse while delegitimizing others. It leaves groups with substantive hopes or concerns out of the debate, unless, for example, metaphysical and theological points can be "translated" into rights and risk language. Evans shows that bioethicists characterize their work not as "translation," but as "clarification" of theologians' "vague" arguments, thereby delegitimating the input of theologians. Bioethicists indeed became more qualified to debate such matters, because they were able to successfully institutionalize formal rationality within bioethics commissions as the only acceptable form of argumentation.

Thus the winners in this decidedly non-neutral arrangement have been bioethicists, scientists, and engineers, who have formed a tacit pact, or what Jonathan Moreno calls "the great bioethics compromise." Bioethicists are given funding in exchange for guaranteeing "science a green light disguised as a flashing yellow" (Moreno 2005, 14). Bioethicists and scientists were able, for example, to secure human genetic engineering as part of their jurisdiction and thus define the debate in terms of the acceptable ends of safety, autonomy, and justice. Others have made similar analyses (e.g., Rosenberg 1999; Stevens 2000; see also Fox and Swazey 2008, 308–9). Indeed, a thin discourse serves the needs of the bureaucratic state more than the public. Bioethicists often serve unelected officials with little public legitimacy. Thus, "the primary consumer of [bioethics] wants it to have a system where values are not up for discussion, and the debate is about the most efficacious means for forwarding those taken-for-granted values" (Evans 2002, 223). As Mark Brown (2008) notes, this is premised on a rationalist view of expertise according to which experts provide value-neutral knowledge that enables citizens to effectively pursue their subjective preferences.

Of course, the problem is that the knowledge is not "value neutral." Instrumentalism emphasizes certain values while concealing others. Thus, in a highly undemocratic fashion, experts constrain dialogue and narrow options without opening up these terms of constraint for debate. The result is a limited, impoverished moral vocabulary that is not representative of the full range of views in a pluralist society or the full moral dimensions of the bioethical issues under debate.[34]

Neutrality or a "view from nowhere" is not an option; substantive questions will be answered one way or another. It is more conducive to an educated citizenry and informed debate to explicitly consider a range of perspectives on these issues, rather than attempt to avoid them or dilute them through abstraction. This calls for a rich framing of bioethical inquiry, one that articulates and evaluates various ends or goods in addition to the means-ends considerations of instrumentalism. As Albert Dzur and Daniel Levin note, "bioethics commissions should be . . . judged successful according to their capacity to facilitate a wider public dialogue over ethical questions in the medical domain rather than by their ability to find the best possible answers to these questions" (Dzur and Levin 2007, 134). Indeed, "education in a democratic polity" may be "the primary function of the social-issue presidential commission" (Flitner 1986, 5; see also Wolanin 1975, 20).

Thus my defense of rich public bioethics stems from a particular understanding of its role within a pluralist democracy (see Dzur and Levin 2004). This role is that of the "public forum," and it is one in which experts neither underachieve by shying away from questions of ends or goods nor overreach by providing default answers to these questions, answers that are not opened up to reasoned, explicit inquiry. Bioethical dilemmas are intertwined with power and conflicts of value, interest, opinion, and worldview. Given this context, public bioethics institutions can best serve the common interest by mobilizing a wide range of intellectual resources[35] to openly articulate and evaluate the positions within these conflicts, thereby enabling citizens to better understand the values and contest the powers at work in the politics of bioethics (Brown 2008).

Evans proposed the creation of an "ends commission" to complement the "means to ends commissions" that contributed to the thinning of public bioethical debate. Kass approvingly cited Evans, claiming that the council's

> first charge is a mandate to raise questions not only about the best means to certain agreed-upon ends, but also about the worthiness of the ends themselves, a mandate to be clear about all of the human

goods at stake that we seek to promote or defend. It is a call to restore to public bioethics the concerns that gave rise to the field in the late 1960s and early 1970s: Where is biotechnology taking us? What does this mean for our humanity? What kind of people do we wish to be, and what sort of a society do we wish to become? We are charged once again to thicken and enrich public bioethics discourse, away from the more limited, explicitly practical approaches adopted by the collaboration of scientists/physicians and professional bioethicists through the work of previous national commissions and regulatory bodies. (Kass 2005, 224–25)

Thus the Kass Council was designed as an experiment in rich public bioethics practicing substantive rationality and adopting a more holistic perspective on the human condition. As a result, it put an end to the "great bioethics compromise" and not surprisingly drew criticisms from many scientists and professional bioethicists. Rather than formulate means-ends procedures, seek consensus, or reduce options to the right answer, the council often multiplied options or simply spurred critical thinking by providing a deep exploration and delineation of a variety of moral perspectives.[36] This offered not only wider representativeness in a pluralist democracy; in providing a rich ethical analysis, it also fostered heightened awareness by its citizens.

Rich Bioethics Is Not Partisan Politics

In opposition to this narrative about enriching public bioethics, many bioethicists, scientists, liberal commentators, and others argued that the Kass Council was fundamentally a partisan body espousing a "conservative" philosophy designed to rubber-stamp the president's predetermined agenda. The first section of this book argues that the Kass Council's version of public bioethics was not fundamentally about partisanship. And it was certainly not, as bioethicist R. Alta Charo (2007) contends, about basing governance on fear, religion, or "morals regulation." Rather, the rich bioethics of the council was about recovering a more adequate picture of being human, a wider, more robust ethical vocabulary, and a more inclusive, explicit public debate. It was a way to politicize bioethics in the sense of engaging diverse publics in matters of ultimate concern. Of course, partisan politics in the negative sense of preventing discussion in order to promote special interests is part of any public bioethics. But this is inimical, certainly not intrinsic, to rich public bioethics.

To reduce the Kass Council to partisanship is to dismiss what was most fundamental and important about its work. In its moral inquiry, the council modeled a version of rich public bioethics in response to the shortcomings inherent in the instrumentalist framing of previous commissions. The instrumentalist approach illuminates certain issues, but it also casts much in shadow, particularly as biomedicine continues to raise questions about the nature of a good life and a good society and not merely right conduct for physicians and medical researchers. As I will argue, the council's own version of rich public bioethics was not perfect, but it did provide a more adequate response to a problem rooted within the modern worldview that was implicitly adopted by previous commissions. The following chapters elucidate this problem and use the Kass Council to demonstrate how a rich public bioethics can mitigate it.

TWO

The Deeper History of the Kass Council

In *The Fundamental Principles of the Metaphysics of Morals* (1785), Immanuel Kant wanted to seek out and establish a foundation for ethics that was based in the autonomy of rational individuals. Kant was compelled to seek out such a foundation anew because values that had once been inscribed in the order of things as guaranteed by God seemed to have lost their footing in light of the scientific findings of Isaac Newton. Kant's solution was to collapse these values into the human will. Although by Kant's account morality required the willing of an autonomous agent, he sought to preserve a universal moral law that could stand as analogous to the universal physical law governing the movement of the heavenly bodies. True, his scheme required that he sunder the subjective from the objective, leaving the subject a radically alien seat of purpose in a world of mechanical laws. But Kant saw his notion of rationality as binding the realm of willing and freedom tightly to the realm of obligation and necessity. He insisted that autonomy means willing the acceptance of, not inventing, the moral law. Yet as Iris Murdoch (1971) points out, it is not a very big step from Kant to the "sovereign becoming" of the Nietzschean self projecting its will onto an indifferent nature. For both, the sovereign moral concept is freedom, ultimately leaving the idea of the good empty, to be filled by human choice.

Thomas Hobbes—responding to religious upheaval with his own "science of man"—had earlier worked out a theory of politics and ethics as human construction. Disaster results when governments take it as their business to perfect souls according to an objective standard. Human inclinations are diverse, according to their diverse customs, constitutions, and opinions. The causes of discord and strife lie less in human failure to seek the good than in their conflicting notions about what the good is. Individuals enter into contract with one another to avoid the violent death typical of the state of nature. The business of government is not to tell us how to live, but to protect our well-being and help us get along justly and peacefully.

Evans is right to note the historical contingencies behind the rise of instrumentalism in public bioethics. It could have worked out otherwise. But it is clear that this outcome runs with the grain of modern thought. When facing an ethical dilemma, we as a society and as individuals just do tend to think in terms of individual rights, risks, and equality.

Any bioethics that did not take rights, risks, and justice into account would be severely flawed. But this is not the entirety of ethics. It is, rather, what T. M. Scanlon (1998) called a "rump morality," or morality understood as principles for what we owe to one other. This rump morality is distinct from "morality in the wider sense," which asks questions about what kinds of lives are good or bad for people to lead. Modern ethics— stemming from Kant and, via the utilitarians, Hobbes—has largely omitted this wider sense, thereby providing a narrow image of humanity (Anscombe 1958). In doing so, it omits many important aspects of the human condition including the meaning of wisdom, friendship, and love, a deep concept of happiness, the meaning of human excellence, procreation, suffering, and mortality, and the fundamental question of how we ought to live.

My defense of rich public bioethics begins with the observation that biomedical science and technology are posing questions about these wider aspects of moral life. These are questions that all members of society must face together. We need to find ways, then, to put this wider ethics into the public forum. Bioethics commissions are good places to do so, because they command a national audience, yet have no policymaking authority. The Kass Council did this kind of "putting back in," a necessary task because instrumental public bioethics does not succeed in avoiding these issues, despite its attempt at a "neutral" framework. Rather, it succeeds only in treating them implicitly, without subjecting assumptions to the light of reasoned analysis.

The move from the realm of obligation (rights) to flourishing (goods) raises questions confronted by the ancients, which is why it is important to leaven the proximal history of the previous chapter with some deep history. To understand the case for a rich bioethics, it is insufficient to look at individual problems (such as human experimentation) posed by science and technology. Rather, we must look at the very way we tend to go about looking, that is, the frames that we bring to bear on these issues, which are themselves fundamentally shaped by the rise of modern science and technology.

This deep history introduces two such frames or myths that are challenged by rich bioethics in ways that I will demonstrate in chapters 3 and 4. I mean by "myth" a story that is widely accepted despite scanty empirical evidence. Both myths come in the form of "great divides." Hobbes introduced the first great divide between self and society, which was thought necessary to secure liberty and fairness by distinguishing an inviolable private sphere pertaining to the (irrational) good from a rational public sphere pertaining to the right. Kant can symbolize the second great divide between the realms of nature and freedom, or body and mind, which was thought necessary to secure human dignity. Where instrumental bioethics implicitly adopts these myths, rich bioethics questions them.

Society can better protect the values that the myths are designed to secure by rejecting the myths and explicitly confronting matters of the good and the embodied whole of human nature. This approach remains truer than instrumentalism to the Enlightenment project of subjecting ends as well as means to the test of reason. Our constitutively social and biological nature grounds much that is necessary for our flourishing. Rich public bioethics is the project of recovering a fuller moral vocabulary in a broadened public forum for exploring the human condition in relation to biomedical and behavioral science and technology.

Ancient Roots of Bioethics

Reflection on what it means to be human, to live an excellent life, and the human capacity to heal and otherwise alter mind, body, and soul predates modern science and the political liberalism that have so thoroughly shaped contemporary bioethics.[1] Indeed, the roots of bioethics reach the two bedrocks of Western culture: Athens and Jerusalem, reason and revelation. Though these ancient roots are diverse, we can extract three essential features that will be of use in characterizing the council's work: (a) the natural or divine order of things as prescribing the proper place of humans within it; (b) ethics as knowledge of this order; and (c) the human self as an integral part of this order. These three aspects of ancient bioethics, then, speak to an understanding of nature, rationality, and the self.

Ethics and Nature

The first two points are best treated together by looking at how Plato and Aristotle understood the nature of ethical inquiry.[2] For both philosophers there was a natural order that existed prior to human conventions. Indeed, philosophy begins when discourse about the gods and the ancestors is replaced with discourse about nature, which transcends any local custom. Their bioethics—and their politics—was first based in a philosophical anthropology, knowing what human nature is. This inquiry led to knowledge of what is best in human nature, and guidelines for cultivating excellence. It is a teleological account of ethics, where understanding what the right action is requires knowing the good, purpose, or "what-for" (*telos*) of the human. Following Aristotle, Alasdair MacIntyre explained *telos* in terms of *function*. For example, a watch and a farmer are both "functional concepts," because "the concept of a watch cannot be defined independently of the concept of a good watch nor the concept of a farmer independently of that of a good farmer" (MacIntyre 1984, 58). He goes on to explain that "moral arguments within the classical, Aristotelian tradition . . . involve at least one central functional concept, the concept of *man* understood as having an essential nature and an essential purpose or function" (MacIntyre 1984, 58). Ethics and political philosophy take their bearing from ends, or what the human can become, rather than how most humans happen to be.[3]

For a teleological style of bioethics, an anthropological investigation into human ends informs a normative understanding about the proper limits of biomedicine. This is apparent in the works of the ancient Greek physician Hippocrates. For Hippocrates, the aim of medicine was "preserving nature, not altering it" ("Precepts," 19), and the physician had an obligation to "refuse to treat those overwhelmed by disease, since in such cases medicine is powerless" ("On *technè*," 3). This ideal of working with nature found further philosophical expression in Aristotle's distinction between cultivation and construction: that is, between the *technai* of agriculture, education, and medicine, which assist nature in the realization of qualities that would appear to some degree independently of human action, versus such *technai* as carpentry, which introduce into nature forms that would not appear without human intervention (see *Physics* II, 1, 193a12–17; *Politics* VII, 17, 1337a2; and *Oeconomica* I, 1, 1342a26–1343b2). The notion of the physician as one who cultivates health with quite limited technical means was allied as well to a paternalistic or authoritarian model of the profession.

As a further example of the ancient understanding of the limits of medicine, Socrates argued against excessive care of the body. He claimed that such care hinders the practice of virtue because an obsessive worry about bodily health distracts one from higher pursuits, especially philosophy and matters of living well (see *Republic*, 406d–407d). Happiness consists in excellence, not in bodily well-being.

For Aristotle, the ultimate end of human life is happiness in the objective sense of well-being, not the fulfillment of whatever one's preferences happen to be. Happiness is an activity of the soul that perfects its highest, or rational, form. For Plato, the just or ideal city would be ruled by philosophers because they pursue true human ends and have the knowledge to educate citizens in these ends. As with Hippocrates, bioethics here is not about respecting individual preferences or rights. It is rather a matter of knowledge and education into the virtues so that we understand what it is to be human and thus how we can flourish. This knowledge is not only or even primarily used for manipulation through technical means. It is knowledge of the human essence, which includes accepting the limits of that form.

Plato and Aristotle reserved only qualified praise for democracy. As their ruling principle is freedom, democracies tend to lose sight of wisdom and excellence, especially when a democratic regime is mixed with an oligarchic one in which the ruling principle is the pursuit of wealth.

Democracy is also suspect because it is based to some degree on the notion that there is no right answer to these ethical and metaphysical questions. We do not decide solutions to arithmetic problems by vote or market dynamics. For the ancients, neither should we decide solutions to moral questions in these ways. We ought to seek the true answers. Though ethical knowledge is not exact in the sense that geometry is, it is a species of knowledge nonetheless (*Nicomachean Ethics* I, 3).[4]

Those who propounded the classic natural-right teaching maintained that the good is essentially different from the pleasant. Humans have a variety of wants, which precede the pleasures and provide the channels within which the pleasures move. The different kinds of wants are not an unorganized bundle of urges. Rather, there is a natural order or hierarchy of the wants, which points back to the constitution of the human. For the ancients, as Leo Strauss explains, "The good life simply, is the life in which the requirements of man's natural inclinations are fulfilled in the proper order to the highest possible degree" (Strauss 1953, 127).

Hellenistic and Roman Stoic philosophers similarly emphasized philosophy as a practice in coming to know the good through a study of human nature and the natural world. The goal of life lies in the selection, through reason, of things according to nature. Some Stoics describe virtues as a kind of science (*epistèmè*) of making these choices well or as an expertise (*technè*) concerned with the whole of life.[5]

During the Middle Ages, articulations of natural-law ethics were enclosed within the framework of revelation, which introduced new virtues (love, hope, and charity) and a new focus on the salvation of the individual's soul. Natural law was reconceived as having been originally created by God—the purposes and laws of nature are God's purposes and divine law. Thus, though different in many ways from the rationalism of ancient Athens, the Hebraic tradition of Jerusalem shares the essential principle that ethics involves knowledge of humans' proper ends and place within a larger order. Applied to bioethical issues, this understanding of ethics would limit the scope of human action. Concerns about playing God that arise in connection with biotechnology speak to this point (cf. Ramsey 1970; Lawler 2002). Humans are creatures, not the Creator; some realms of being such as procreation are given or gifted and thus are improper places for human design. This principle can also be seen to refer to mortality. For example, a passage from Psalms reads: "Teach us to number our days that we may gain a heart of wisdom" (Ps. 90:10–12), which Lawrence Vogel (2006) interprets as a claim that medicine should not become a Promethean effort to eliminate imperfection or extend life at all costs. Similarly, Kass argues that the sin of Babel was that its residents aspired to self-re-creation through their arts and crafts (Kass 2003).[6] Kass (1991) also notes that biblical resources are available to critique advocates of euthanasia, especially in the value of suffering as a way to realize our divine-like nature (see Hyde 2001).

Like Plato and Aristotle, the Bible teaches the wisdom of limiting emphasis on the body, in part because this distracts from higher pursuits. Christian intellectual C. S. Lewis warned of the human tendency to be seduced by "the sweet poison of the false infinite" (Lewis 1965, 81). The project to reprogram body and mind is "false" because it misconstrues humans as infinitely pliable rather than as beings with a proper form that constitutes their good. It is a distraction from the art of diligently cultivating one's given nature, which is a quest that is at some point cheapened, rather than advanced, by technical interventions.

Tied to this teleological account of ethos in ancient bioethical thought is an account of *bios*, or life. For the vast majority of ancient cultures, life was accepted as the primary state of things. To be was to be alive. Thus nature displayed everywhere the purposive qualities associated with living organisms. Though certainly available as a kind of metaphysics (e.g., Democritus' atoms in the void) for the ancients, the predominant modern image of a lifeless, mechanical, objective universe set in opposition to the human soul was simply not widely accepted. Rather, the problem facing panvitalism was to explain death, which was the apparent negation of the natural and intelligible order of things. This explains the power of the death motif from the beginnings of human thought (see Jonas 1966).

The Ancient Self and Community

Teleological ethics clearly ties the self to nature. But humans, more than any creature, have a nature that is in need of or in potency to culture. They become whole only through their material and ideational cultures. Thus, the ancients also had a notion of the self that is constitutively social. Since it is reason or speech that distinguishes humans from other animals and since speech is communication, "humanity itself is sociality" (Strauss 1953, 129). Affection, friendship, and love are as natural to humans as concern with their own self-interests. Furthermore, this radical sociality means that the perfection of human nature includes the greatest social virtue, justice.

In the *Republic*, Socrates argued that the just or ideal polis would need to move beyond political ideology into the management of marriage, family, and procreation.[7] Similarly, in the *Politics* Aristotle argued that the whole, the polis, exists prior to the parts, individuals, and that the parts can only be understood in their relation to the whole. The whole is that for the sake of which the parts exist and in which they find meaning. Yet Aristotle was also the first critic to argue that Plato's solution to the strife born of diversity within the polis goes too far. In seeking to harmonize the polis, Plato nearly reduces it to a homogenous body by doing away with even the most private sphere of procreative and familial relations. Aristotle rejoins that although the polis does precede any given individual, its raison d'être is to serve the good life for the citizen.

The ancient self is also an embodied soul.[8] In a way similar to Plato's metaphor of the rational soul as the charioteer guiding the passions (*Phaedrus*), Aristotle argues that the soul rules the body by despotism. By this he means that the faculties of the body merely experience pleasure and pain, seeking the former and avoiding the latter. The rational part of the soul instructs the body that it is sometimes preserved by what is painful and destroyed by what is pleasurable. One who responds merely to the demands of the body, like a child, cannot be reasoned with and must be ruled by force or deception. Over time one's passions can be ruled over more reasonably as one learns to discipline and tailor them to appropriate circumstances.

In his discussion of the art of wealth making in the *Politics*, Aristotle criticizes the excessive pursuit of commodious luxury. Indeed he seems to portray the root of injustice as the abolition of limits on the desires of the body. The resulting excess focuses too much attention on leading mere life (*zoe*) (i.e., fulfilling bodily necessities) rather than leading the good life (*bios*) (i.e., cultivating the rational faculty). Pursuing the good life requires leisure time, which for Aristotle is afforded to those wealthy enough to own "natural slaves," who are marked "from the hour of their birth" for subjection (*Politics*, I, 5).

The Roman Stoics also dealt with bioethical issues stemming from notions of the self. They maintained that one must strive to be free of the passions, which engender suffering. The Stoics sought freedom in the "knowing consent to the meaningful necessity of the whole" (Jonas 1966, 221). Many Stoics were influenced by Epicurus' rank-ordering of human desires and his insight regarding the foolishness of seeking those "unnecessary" pleasures that increase rather than limit wants. A further implication of this philosophy is that one who approaches death with right reason will accept it calmly, with freedom from the passions.

Transition to Modernity

Both scripture and ancient political thought, then, work in a moral language of virtue, character, purpose, and discipline that instructs about the proper human form and ends. They instruct limits to the pursuit of technical self-intervention and bodily desires. Yet both revelation and reason have been taken to the opposite conclusion, foreshadowing disagreements within contemporary bioethics about the proper reach of human power.

For example, some scholars challenge interpretations of the Bible as counseling limitations to human action. This dispute can be seen in the two founding theological figures in bioethics. The Episcopalian Joseph Fletcher tended toward a rights-based embrace of technology, while the Methodist Paul Ramsey tended toward a restrictive approach: "Ramsey interprets God's *agape* in a way radically distinct from Fletcher's interpretation: it does not will humankind's good, but commands humankind's obedience" (Jonsen 1998, 48). This disagreement taps into arguments about how to interpret the scriptural meaning of humans as "co-creators." A Psalm reads, "I say, 'You are gods'" (Ps. 82:6).[9]

The Catholic interpretation of co-creation holds that humans ought to strive for recapturing the likeness of God,[10] but through prayer and acts of charity, not primarily through physical manipulations of the world or the body. Some heterodox interpretations of scripture argue that humans ought to take other measures, including magic and technology, to recapture the likeness of God. This approach, which might best be called "gnostic," condones a wider embrace of biomedical technology. The gnostic standpoint recurs throughout Christian history, viewing the human soul as bound by the moral law of the natural order, but the human spirit as authentically free of any objective dictates. Thus it rejects the notion of a definable human nature, which would subject sovereign existence to a predetermined essence. Spiritual human existence does not belong to an objective scheme. It is a law unto itself and freely shaped by the powers of human knowledge. Thus, the primary function of knowledge is reconceptualized not as receptivity[11] or contemplation (*theoria*), but as manipulation (*technè*).

The gnostic view never gained widespread support, in part because its magic was never very effective in achieving the transformations sought. But views similar to those of gnosticism gained wider acceptance in the aftermath of the Protestant reformation of the sixteenth century. Indeed, they were often utilized by the early modern founders of the new natural sciences to cast their work in theological, and thus more culturally acceptable, terms. For example, Francis Bacon wrote:

> For man by the fall fell at the same time from his state of innocency and from his dominion over creation. Both of these losses however can even in this life be in some part repaired; the former by religion and faith, the latter by arts and sciences. For creation was not by the curse made altogether and forever a rebel, but in virtue of that charter "In the sweat of thy face shall thou eat bread," it is now by various labors (not certainly by disputations or idle magical ceremonies, but by various labors) at length and in some measure subdued to the supplying of man with bread, that is, to the uses of human life. (*Novum Organum* 1620, LII)

The new scientific method was a more effective means to fulfill the human calling toward perfection. But "perfection" took on a radically different, more aimless meaning under the modern worldview, devoid as it was of any natural telos.

The Rise of Modernity

When Niccolò Machiavelli promoted "new modes and orders" unlike those which had previously existed, he was expressing a vision that came to define modernity (from the late Latin "modernus," derivative of the classical

Latin "modo," meaning "just now" or "in a certain manner"). This vision was shared by others such as Bacon, Galileo Galilei, René Descartes, and Isaac Newton. These thinkers were partly motivated by the old aim of natural theology, as Johannes Kepler phrased it, "to think God's thoughts after him," perhaps limiting the role of God but keeping Him central to morality. Yet, from politics and science to philosophy and religion these thinkers also argued for the possibility of introducing a radical historical break. From the Renaissance through the Enlightenment traditional restraints were replaced with an ethical commitment to the pursuit of technology.

In its basic understandings of nature, rationality, and the self, the moderns differed radically from the premoderns. The old way of thinking about these issues was challenged by the ideas that: (a) nature is a nonpurposive collection of "facts" and therefore can provide no moral guidance; (b) ends or "values" are thus reduced from a species of knowledge to personal preferences projected upon a mechanistic world; and (c) the human self is best conceived as a pre-social and autonomous subject.

Science and Nature

First, modern science altered what it means to *know*—from an understanding of knowledge as contemplation of a thing's nature to the ability to control the thing. In the preface to *The Great Instauration* (1620), Bacon first made the radical argument that "human knowledge and human power meet in one." Complaining of the vain speculations of the ancients, Bacon urged "that knowledge be used not as a courtesan, for pleasure and vanity only . . . but as a spouse for generation, fruit, and comfort." The production of knowledge would culminate in "the conquest of nature for the relief of man's estate" (*Novum Organum*, LII). This mindset is "technological" at its core, as it upholds an intimate alliance between knowing and changing the world: "the nature of things betrays itself more readily under the vexations of art than in its natural freedom" (Bacon, "Plan of the Work," paragraph 21).[12] This leads to a focus on manipulating the world "out there" rather than transforming the inner worlds of wants, needs, and desires.[13]

Second, this altered notion of knowledge changed the human relation to and understanding of nature, including human nature. Descartes argued, "So soon as I had acquired some general notions concerning Physics . . . I believed that I could not keep them concealed without greatly sinning against the law which obliges us to procure, as much as in us lies, the general good of all mankind." He continued that new knowledge can

render ourselves the masters and possessors of nature. This is not merely to be desired with a view to the invention of an infinity of arts and crafts which enable us to enjoy without any trouble the fruits of the earth and all the good things which are to be found there, but also principally because it brings about the preservation of health, which is without doubt the chief blessing and foundation of all other blessings in this life. For the mind depends so much on the tempera-ment and disposition of the bodily organs that, if it is possible to find a means of rendering men wiser and cleverer than they have hitherto been, I believe that it is in medicine that it must be sought. (*Discourse on Method* 1637, VI)

Descartes upheld science and technology as tools of a this-worldly salva-tion, where it would be a sin *not* to eat more from the tree of knowledge. Both he and Bacon—working from this altered understanding of knowl-edge and nature—exalt the preservation of bodily health, treating it as an infinite project, rather than seeing it as one, limited, good among many, as the ancients had done.

Third, modern scientific knowledge rejects explanations in terms of ends or purposes. Bacon ridiculed the Aristotelian science of final causes:

[F]or although the most general principles in nature ought to be held merely positive, as they are discovered, and cannot with truth be referred to a cause, nevertheless the human understanding being unable to rest still seeks something prior in the order of nature. And then it is that in struggling toward that which is further off it falls back upon that which is nearer at hand, namely, on *final causes, which have relation clearly to the nature of man rather than to the nature of the uni-verse;* and from this source have strangely defiled philosophy. (*Novum Organum,* XLVIII, emphasis added)

Science, the only true rationality, reveals objective facts. Descartes was among the first to set thinking toward the complementary notion that ends are subjective and are thus not properly considered objects of knowledge. For example, in *Discourse on Method*, he extolled mathematics "because of the certainty and self-evidence of the way it reasons" (I). By contrast, he writes, "I compared the writings on morality of the ancient pagans with the very magnificent and superb palaces that were built only on sand and mud. They very much extol the virtues and make them appear more valuable than anything else in the world; but they do not provide adequate instruction about how to recognize them, and frequently something that they classify as virtue is merely insensibility, pride, despair or parricide" (I). Descartes saw philosophy as a tradition consisting of doubt and dispute, concluding "that it was impossible that anything solid could have been built on foundations that were so weak" (I). The new natural sciences, by contrast, promised certainty that could ground progress.[14]

But it is Isaac Newton who best symbolizes the triumph of a mechanistic, mathematical universe, understandable without recourse to final ends. Yet Newton found it difficult not to believe in a divine artificer. Indeed, he saw in gravity the constant hand of God at operation in the universe. Later interpreters such as Pierre Laplace began to distance God from the operations of the heavenly bodies, first through deism and later through more thoroughly mechanistic accounts. In a reversal of ancient epistemology and ontology, the modern mathematicization of nature held that intelligibility meant reducibility to the most elemental. At its core, modern science does not explain phenomena in terms of causes, but rather provides a descriptive account of quantitative constants in different positions along a time series. Any rational properties of such a series (e.g., a planetary orbit) were no longer understood as having an intrinsic reason or as aspiring toward harmony. Rather, they were the mechanical uniformity of the elemental factors involved (see Jonas 1966).

The a-purposive account of the world was extended to living things, including humans, through Charles Darwin's theory on evolution through natural selection, published in 1859. This new understanding of life opened up new powers for healing and altering the human organism. Yet just as these new powers were gained, traditional sources of order were being eroded. After Darwin, there no longer seemed to be an objective vision of the human form or divine or natural order to direct the newfound technological powers. The original essence of humanity, the form that the ancients

believed to provide standards of excellence attainable through right reasoning and proper training, seemed to evaporate into the transience of the
evolutionary process.

For modern science, unlike ancient thought, the absence of life is the
primary state of being. Thus, the problem was how to explain life in terms
of non-life, by reducing it to its physical and chemical properties. The ancient monism of life-as-being-as-good had been sundered into a dualism
most cogently put forward by Descartes in his split between the mind
(*res cogitans*) and the body (*res extensa*). This unstable dualism was eventually resolved into the modern doctrines of materialism and idealism.[15]
As Hans Jonas explained:

> The very possibility of an "inanimate universe" emerged as the
> counterpart to the increasingly exclusive stress laid on the *human*
> soul, on its inner life and its incommensurability with anything in
> nature. The fateful divorce, stretched to the point of a complete for-
> eignness which left nothing in common between the parted mem-
> bers, henceforth qualified them both by this mutual exclusion. As the
> retreating soul drew about itself all spiritual significance and meta-
> physical dignity, contracting them and itself alike within its inner-
> most being, it left the world divested of all such claims and, though
> at first decidedly demonic, in the end indifferent to the very question
> of value either way. (Jonas 1966, 13–14)

Modern science sundered the realms of freedom and nature, posing a challenge to ethics. Absent a purposeful natural order as a normative guide,
the question for ethics became: What are the grounds for the justification
of norms and for distinguishing lower and higher pleasures?

Modern Ethics and Politics

Modern ethics offered three main responses to the removal of a religious
or normative transcendent order. First, in his formulation of the autonomous self Kant salvaged human dignity in a Newtonian world. In self-
governance, he also found a way to abandon the religious morality of obedience, which he saw as another threat to individual dignity. Rational

autonomy as the source of moral knowledge meant that all rational adults are capable of discerning right from wrong. It is thus the basis for justifying the view that we each can rightly claim to direct our own actions without interference from those with supposedly superior wisdom (see Schneewind 1998). For Kant, "autonomy . . . is the basis of the dignity of human and of every rational nature" (*Fundamental Principles of the Metaphysics of Morals* 1785, II). Kant and others on the European continent such as Jean-Jacques Rousseau grounded ethics in reason and pictured it less as human construction than as antecedent condition.

Second, and by contrast, Thomas Hobbes, John Locke, and others in England conceived of ethics as based in pleasure and pain and pictured political morality as a human construction. Both Hobbes and Locke aspired to match Newtonian atomism with an atomistic science of humanity. Far from being Aristotle's political animals, individual humans are not "by nature" political. Rather they predate society and sacrifice some of their power for the safety and comforts that political community affords. This tradition gave rise to the ethical theory of utilitarianism. Like Kant, John Stuart Mill attempted to salvage an objective account of the good that allowed for judgments about their relative quality. He did so, however, by appealing to experience rather than a priori principles (*Utilitarianism*, 1863 II). Yet just as Kantian autonomy has largely been transformed into the much more subjectivist "individual autonomy,"[16] so too utilitarianism— via mainstream capitalism—has become a theory of preference satisfaction.[17] In both cases, then, the object is to respect and satisfy the desires of individuals.

The third response is the emphasis of Friedrich Nietzsche and, later on, existentialists such as Jean-Paul Sartre on the human will. The implications of science call for "the re-valuation of all values." The consequences of truthfulness in science and morality force us to face the implications of a meaningless universe. The modern worldview necessitates that "*the highest values devaluate themselves.* The aim is lacking: 'why?' finds no answer . . . We lack the least right to posit a beyond or in-itself of things that might be 'divine' or morality incarnate" (Nietzsche 1967, preface, I, 2–3). Each individual should mold his or her own values as the pure expression of selfhood, ignoring what society, in its staid fashion, calls good and evil. Nietzsche argued that Kant's deontology and Mill's utilitarianism (not to mention Christianity) had no foundations and were themselves manifestations of the will to power.

To restate the fundamental transformation in the science of ethics: Both Aristotle and Mill describe action as for the sake of some end. But for Aristotle the end is understood as a potency inherent in the nature of the entity that performs the action and in its cosmic context, whereas for Mill the end is simply an actor's subjective preference. For Aristotle, the model is the exercise of an ability that realizes or perfects that ability; virtues realize or perfect human nature analogous to the way health perfects the body. For Mill, the model is more like a commercial transaction; virtues are those actions in which benefits exceed costs. The end result is that, with Nietzsche and much contemporary moral sentiment, "The good life does not consist, as it did according to the earlier notion, in compliance with a pattern antedating the human will, but consists primarily in originating the pattern itself" (Strauss 1989, 244). Modern individuals thus tend to see themselves as managers of life projects. This calls forth feelings of both responsibility and moral uncertainty: "If my life is a project, what exactly is the purpose of the project? How do I tell a successful project from a failure?" (Elliott 2003, 299).

All three modern ethical traditions similarly move individual freedom to the fore of any political or economic project. Though liberal economists such as Adam Smith and David Riccardo recognized the primacy of production over politics, they seeded mainstream capitalist theories that conceived of the techno-economic order as fundamentally separate from politics, that is, as an emergent order of individual preference expression. Karl Marx rebelled against just this point, arguing that the technological productive forces of the economy have more influence over human life than any political institution and should be subjected to democratic controls. The triumph of capitalism reinforced a commonsense notion that technology is a value-neutral realm divorced from politics and governed instead by the invisible hand of demand and supply.

Disembedded from ethics and politics, industrial capitalism unleashed the inherently infinite growth of the consumerist desires of the *animal laborans* (Arendt 1958). Yet this also received ethical justification from Locke, who emancipated acquisitiveness by equating true charity with unlimited appropriation without concern for the needs of others. Indeed, since reason cannot control the passions, only another passion (i.e., self-interest) can do so. Thus the art of wealth making in commerce was transformed from an activity that was at best ethically tolerated into a true calling (Hirschman 1977).

The early moderns sought ways to cope with conflicts brought about by the age of exploration, sectarian wars, and industrialism. Abstractions such as Hobbes's and Locke's "state of nature" helped secure respect for persons and social peace. The laws of their contractual societies were not meant to show the way to one's best self; they were simply meant to limit quarrels. They introduced what Mark Lilla (2007) called "the great separation" between the political order and the divine nexus of God–humans–nature.

Where the ancients took humans as they could be, the moderns took them as they are.[18] In the pre-liberal tradition, politics aspired not only to help make people safe and prosperous, but also to help make them virtuous. By contrast, Hobbes flatly stated "there is no such *Finis ultimis* (utmost ayme,) nor *Summum bonum* (greatest Good,) as is spoken of in the Books of the old Morall Philosophers" (*Leviathan* 1651, XI, 1). Modern liberalism overturned the classical tradition by rejecting its aspirations to "make men moral," arguing instead that this violated fundamental principles of justice and human rights (see George 1993). Founders of the liberal tradition argued that the ancients failed because they aimed too high and based their theories on indefensible considerations of humans' higher goods rather than their actual desires. Machiavelli distinguishes between "the actual truth of matters" and the imaginary republics and princedoms "which have never in fact been seen or known to exist" (*The Prince* 1532, XV). In the opening of his *Tractatus Theologico-Politicus* (1670) Benedict Spinoza attacks the philosophers who conceive humans not as they are but rather as they wish them to be. Such works helped lead to a view in which individual desires are the given, and the task of politics as well as economics is to accommodate them.[19]

Political liberalism is grounded in a very sensible move, as Kwame Appiah (2005) notes, to "leave as much out" of politics as possible. Locke and Hobbes formulated their theories in response to conflict, or in contemporary parlance, in response to values pluralism and multiculturalism. Different metaphysical and religious positions inevitably breed disagreement and often violence. It is best to consider such matters private and construct a society founded on tolerance that can support many views of the good. This position was formulated best by Mill in his harm principle: "[T]he only purpose for which power can be rightfully exercised over any member of a civilized community, against his will, is to prevent harm to others. His own good, either physical or moral, is not a sufficient warrant. He cannot rightfully be compelled to do or forbear because it will be better for him to do so, because it will make him happier, because, in the opinion of others, to do so would be wise or even right" (*On Liberty* 1859, I).

The public sphere, then, is limited to the protection of rights, and the state is otherwise neutral with respect to questions of how best to live. Seeking to summarize and critique liberalism, C. B. Macpherson developed a multifaceted notion of "possessive individualism": (a) what makes us human is freedom from dependence on the wills of others; (b) this means we only form self-interested relations with others; (c) the individual is the proprietor of his own person; (d) each individual's freedom can rightfully be limited only by the obligations necessary to secure the freedom of others; and (e) society consists of a series of market relations (see Macpherson 1962, 263–64).

Though Macpherson captures much that is central to liberalism, his is only one of myriad voices composing the tradition. Indeed, as Appiah notes, the fruit of the early modern theorists is a robust liberal tradition that is "not so much a body of doctrine as a set of debates" (Appiah 2005, ix). These debates are about who we are, who we ought to be, and the nature of a good society. They have shaped contemporary bioethics as well as politics.

The Impact of Modernity on Bioethics

Humiliated after World War I, many young Weimar Protestants were susceptible to the messianic spirit calling for a new ideology to transform the world. The resulting atrocities committed by the Nazi regime reinforced— in politics at large and in bioethics—a commitment to the two myths of the great divides between body (nature) and mind (rational will) and between self (private, goods) and society (public, rights). First, any claims about a human essence or nature not grounded simply in universal reason seemed too easily misused to support notions that some peoples are

naturally inferior, others naturally superior. Second, a government justifying actions from substantive claims about the good life easily slides into
tyranny. Additionally, the Nuremburg Code's demand for international
consensus sent professional and public bioethics along a course toward
universal and secular principles of respect for persons.

This brings the narrative back to the previous chapter and the argument that only an instrumental, thin bioethics is compatible with modern pluralistic liberalism. This view can now be given further consideration. The early moderns adopted a thoroughgoing skepticism concerning
the ability to reason about the good. Reason is only instrumental in nature, helping humans achieve their ends, but not clarifying which ends
are best. In addition to this epistemic claim is the Hobbesian ethical argument for separating matters of the good from politics: the blending of
the two inevitably culminates in violence, in part because there is no reasonable way to settle such fundamental differences. Thus modern liberalism envisioned political association not as the common quest for higher
goods, but as a set of rules and procedures for adjudicating different demands within a framework of rights that is supposedly neutral on substantive questions of the good. Instrumentalism recapitulates this thesis:
public bioethics is not a matter of rationally evaluating different visions of
the good, but of ensuring that the rights of individuals are protected.

In *The Foundations of Bioethics,* Tristram Engelhardt Jr. argues that
this is the only form of public bioethics a pluralist society can legitimately
support. He divides human relations within pluralist modern society into
two types: moral friends and moral strangers. Moral friends belong to a
community, which is "a body of men and women bound together by common moral traditions and/or practices around a shared vision of the good
life" (Engelhardt 1996, 7).[20] They share a "content-full morality," which
provides "sufficient moral premises or rules of evidence and inference to
resolve moral controversies by sound rational argument" and/or "a common commitment to individuals or institutions in authority to resolve
moral controversies" (7). Moral strangers, by contrast, belong to *society,*
which is "an association that compasses individuals who find themselves
in diverse moral communities" (7). They do not share a content-full morality and are left with a "purely procedural morality in which persons
convey to common endeavors the moral authority of their consent" (7).

Within a community, moral friends can rationally work out the right decision with a view toward how it advances their shared understanding of the good life. Within a society, this type of rationality is not available: "The good life does not consist of both a what and a how, but only a how" (Strauss 1989, 244).

For Engelhardt, "there is no content-full bioethics outside of a particular moral perspective" (Engelhardt 1996, 9). In contemporary pluralist societies, each person has his or her personal or cultural biases about what is better and worse, higher and lower, nobler and baser, etc., but these are mere perspectives and thus oftentimes incommensurable: there are no transcendent standards of rationality by which to judge the claims of different communities and persons. Anne Maclean makes a similar claim, that "opposing moral beliefs, opinions, judgements or attitudes may both — or all — be adequate from the standpoint of reason or rationality; indeed, that there need be in such cases *no* standpoint which is *the* standpoint of reason or rationality" (Maclean 1993, 6). Engelhardt realizes that the failure to ground the objectivity of morality brings us to "the brink of nihilism." How are we to justify ethical claims if all substantive ethical statements are relative to a particular tradition? Engelhardt admits, "Blind to final purposes, we turn to ourselves for meaning. As moral strangers, within the fabric of secular morality, we confront godlike choices with impoverished human vision, and without ultimate guideposts" (Engelhardt 1996, 411).[21] Preference satisfaction is the only standard of right action: "*what people want* is the ultimate measure of right and wrong" (Maclean 1993, 10). Though he is not satisfied with his own answer (due to his Christian beliefs), Engelhardt concludes that an instrumental public bioethics is the only possible framework a secular pluralist society can support: "Because there are no decisive secular arguments to establish that one concrete view of the moral life is better morally than its rivals, and since all have not converted to a single moral viewpoint, secular moral authority is the authority of consent" (Engelhardt 1996, 68). Given the plurality and incommensurability of visions of the good life, "all one can say is that one should be sure that the means . . . will produce the desired goals without significant, undesired side effects" (417). This is the argument for instrumental public bioethics.

In the remainder of part I, I will make my case against this argument, maintaining that it is both legitimate and important for our pluralist society to host a substantive conversation, and that, with their high level of prestige and visibility and low level of power, bioethics committees are good locations for this activity.

This conversation is important because the current biomedical revolution is offering new powers that call for a wisdom that considers not just risks and rights but also the question of what it is to lead a humanly meaningful life. Indeed, with its "spiritual hunger" and "progress paradox," the technologically affluent world is crying out for such understanding (Lane 2000; Myers 2000; Easterbrook 2003). With our material success has come the moral weakness of sullenness when it comes to human flourishing—more pleasure, less happiness (Borgmann 2006). We are the "worried well," mastered by new fears and desires rather than being satisfied with the bounties technology offers. Rousseau had already diagnosed this "unintended consequence" of technology. Writing about those who began to procure for themselves the conveniences and commodities afforded by technology, Rousseau claims that "not only did these men proceed to lull both body and mind; through habitual use these conveniences also lost almost all their pleasurableness, degenerating into genuine needs, and the deprivation of them became much more painful than the possession of them was pleasing; and people were unhappy in losing them without being happy in possessing them" (*Discourse on the Origin and Foundations of Inequality* 1754, II).

In order for modernity to be adequate to the challenges that its very successes have wrought, society must openly confront ultimate ends and human goods. Naturally, it is here that reasonable people can disagree. Hobbes and Engelhardt supposed that either violence or tyranny is all that could come of this disagreement. Engelhardt is willing to accept the lesser of two evils—in his mind, a democratic yet overly permissive (even nihilistic) society is better than a virtuous yet authoritarian one. But I will argue that rich public bioethics forges a middle way between these extremes, one in which substantive debate produces the enhanced moral insight and imagination of a wiser and more virtuous democratic polis.

Substantive disagreements occur in the public sphere all the time, though they are often masked behind the supposedly neutral language of science (cf. Frodeman 2003). To suppose that global climate change, for example, is a technical or scientific issue is to miss the elephant in the room—human desires or "lifestyle choices." As with environmental ethics, in bioethics we cannot avoid questions of what it is to live well. We cannot scrub away the substance to arrive at pure procedure (whether by tallying costs and benefits or by ensuring informed consent), because modern science and technology themselves, as well as the utility maximizer and the autonomous subject, are predicated on deeply metaphysical presumptions about who we are, what nature is, and how the two relate. These issues can only be confronted in a more or a less reasonable and explicit fashion. Our future will be decided one way or another. A truly liberal society will avail itself of open eyes, open dialogue, and a full ethical palette. After all, now that a strong liberal tradition is in place, disagreement need not be destructive. It can in fact be productive of a deeper understanding. This is the promise of a rich public bioethics.

THREE

In Defense of Rich Public Bioethics I

Self and Society

Facing imminent death for his crime against Athens, Socrates is visited in prison by his friend Crito, who implores him to escape. In considering possible reasons that could justify fleeing, Socrates sets himself into an imaginary conversation with the laws of Athens. The laws argue that no state can endure if its decisions have no power and are overthrown by individual citizens. Socrates replies that in his case their decision was unjust. The laws retort: "Was there provision for this in the agreement between you and us, Socrates? Or did you undertake to abide by whatever judgments the state pronounced?" Socrates is astonished, but the laws continue: "Since you have been born and brought up and educated, can you deny, in the first place, that you were our child and servant, both you and your ancestors?" (*Crito,* 50c–e).

Socrates paints a complex picture of the relationship between the individual and the polis. At least in democratic Athens, it involves choices and conscious agreements made by citizens with the state. But this is not the entirety of the relationship, because the state is the parent of its citizens. It is the author of their being and education, generating their very existence and fundamentally shaping their identity.

With their parables of the state of nature, Hobbes, Locke, and other early moderns greatly simplified the story of the individual self and his or her society. Human individuals are pre-social beings with their interests fully formed. Through conscious agreements, they construct society. It is they who generate the state, not the other way around. Such social contract theories were motivated by the need to ensure greater individual freedoms. The religious wars of the age revealed the atrocities that can result when Socrates' communalistic vision is pressed too far. Individuals become mere grist for the mills of power and ideology.

For the moderns, the role of the state is reduced from shaper of souls to protector of atomistic rights-bearers. Political association is not about achieving a definite vision of the good life, but about establishing a fair, open framework in which multiple visions can coexist. Liberalism, according to this view, gives a procedural answer to the question of the good: let individuals be free to decide on their own. As long as the conditions of informed consent obtain, the individual is fully in control of developing his or her life plan. Because individuals enter into only voluntary relations, their substantive decisions about what constitutes a good life can be treated as private preferences. Within the neutral framework proffered by government, anyone is free either to consent to or to refuse a proposed contract that would commit them to a certain way of living.

With its overbearing emphasis on reducing risks and ensuring informed consent, instrumentalist public bioethics recapitulates the contractual image of society. Just as the task of government is to remain neutral on matters of the good, so too the task for public bioethics—a small appendage of government—is to ensure a neutral, fair framework in which individuals have the right to make their own choices. The fear in both cases is that the only other alternative is a coercive paternalism in which "the laws" forcibly impose a pattern of existence or a way of life on individuals.

But there is a problem. Humans are not bundles of fully-formed preferences who preexist social and political relations. Socrates' more complex picture is truer to the human condition in which we are thrown into a world that nurtures and shapes us. Oftentimes our own identity and sense of the good can be opaque to ourselves, and we rely on our social surroundings to inform us about who we are and what we want, even if we come to realize that what we want is to be something different than what we see around us.

An important result of our constitutive interdependence is that many of our "personal" decisions about how to live cannot be cordoned off to a private sphere that consists in voluntary contractual relations. My choice to lead a lifestyle that is energy- and materials-intensive has ramifications for others, including future generations. But here the picture gets even more complex, because this is not entirely "my choice." In the U.S., for example, many people effectively have no other choice but to drive cars. We exist within a social context, shaped in part by governmental laws, that greatly influences and in some cases even determines the life choices available to us.

So too, the image of a "neutral" public bioethics is an illusion — "neutrality" is in fact only one way of looking at the human situation. It is undoubtedly an appropriate mode of evaluating the contractual scenarios of human-subjects research where respect for autonomy and the avoidance of harm are of overriding importance. But humans are more than simply rights-bearers and physical harm is not the only threat to their flourishing. Much of human life involves formative relations of care where protecting rights, though important, is only one aspect of the moral picture.

Instrumental bioethics, like the "state of nature" or John Rawls's "veil of ignorance," is a conceptual lens that frames moral language in determinate ways. Autonomous, rights-bearing individuals concerned to avoid harm are set in the foreground, but at the expense of casting in shadow the moral tapestry of the relationships that form our common lifeworld and constitute our selves. These rich aspects of being human are continuously at work in bioethics debates. But the frame provided by instrumentalism conceals them from conscious reflection. As a result, we stumble to work only with the limited moral vocabulary of rights and risks and the truncated mindset of thinking in terms of isolated, ad hoc "problems" to be "fixed."

This creates a need for a rich public bioethics, one that does not replace instrumentalism, but rather restricts this mode of ethical evaluation to its proper sphere and complements it where it falls short. Rich bioethics sheds light where instrumentalism casts shadow; it spurs discussion and expands moral imagination where instrumentalism offers silence and a stunted sense of being human.

In this chapter, I will elaborate on this story regarding the need for a rich public bioethics, a need that stems from the failure of two neutrality theses—one about technology and the other about the state. Moreover, I will argue not only that rich public moral inquiry is compatible with liberal democracy, but that in fostering enhanced individual understanding it is better than instrumentalism at promoting liberal ideals. Two Kass Council reports will provide concrete examples of the way rich public bioethics works and how it is an improvement over instrumentalism.

The Non-Neutrality of Technology with Respect to the Good

The contractual presuppositions of instrumentalism rely on an implicit theory of technology as value neutral. But this is a bad theory, which renders the contractual image of society and its claims about the possibility of privatizing the good highly suspect. A better understanding of how technology works to pattern self and society demonstrates the need for a rich public bioethics capable of explicitly articulating and evaluating the substantive dimensions of our personal and collective decisions.

Instrumentalism understands technologies in means-ends fashion—they are tools that perform set functions. A microwave warms food, a birth-control pill prevents pregnancy, and an automobile transports people. According to this view, technologies only embed values of effectiveness with respect to a given function. They are otherwise neutral with respect to the wider practices and contexts in which they are employed. They can be put to good or bad uses by good or bad people. This instrumentalist view of technology is a necessary condition for any contractual view of modern society. If artifacts fulfill only narrowly defined functions, then personal, corporate, and public decisions about their development and use will not have any broader impacts on society and the human lifeworld. These decisions, then, can be treated as isolated contractual agreements. The sole task for governments, including public bioethics, is to ensure that these contracts are respectful of the rights of the parties involved.

Yet as Martin Heidegger (1954) put it, this understanding of technology, though "correct," is not "true." Philosophers of technology are nearly unanimous in conceiving of technology as non-neutral. Technological artifacts, knowledge, and systems are far more than intended functions. Winner (2004), for example, proposed thinking of technologies as "forms of life." As artifacts become enrolled into social and personal

processes, they come to life as morally significant actors shaping the social order, personal relationships, goals, hopes, and fears—in short, de-
limiting and structuring the channels available to pursue a good life and
influencing conceptions of what a good life is.

Microwaves do not just heat food; they restructure daily life, including
family meals, and impact agriculture and economy. The introduction of
the birth-control pill did not just enhance contraceptive efficacy; it played
a role in the radical social upheavals of the 1960s and 1970s, including
women's liberation and changing conceptions about sexuality, gender,
and family. Automobiles do not just transport people in an otherwise unchanged world; they shape infrastructures, create markets, alter residen-
tial patterns and communities, and influence, through their use of oil and
other materials, international relations and the global environment. Light
bulbs do not merely illuminate previously existing spaces, but make possible new spaces with new practices. The cumulative effect of modern
medicine is not just cures for individuals, but an aging population, including many people undergoing prolonged periods of diminishment neces-
sitating care. The movable-type printing press did far more than mass-
produce books and pamphlets; it contributed to religious and political
upheaval and shifts in self-identity as typographic thinking replaced oral
thinking.

According to the neutral view of technology, the good is privatized
and presumed to be freely chosen by individuals wholly in ownership and
control of their persons. But the impacts of technology cannot be so easily
privatized and controlled. Indeed, the technological patterning of life occurs in a way that no one freely chooses. You cannot be without voice mail
or email, at least not without severe consequences; the experience of wilderness is attenuated by others' cell phones, even if you do not have one;
and we all feel the impacts of global climate change regardless of what car
we do or do not drive. In addition, major technological systems from water
treatment plants to interstate highways to electricity grids structure the lifeworld in determinate ways, making possible certain activities while fore-
closing others. Technologies promote and discourage ways of life in ways
that no individual can control or direct through contracts.

Biomedical enhancements are a textbook case of supposedly private
decisions with substantive consequences for others. Proponents of liberal
eugenics, for example, argue that parents ought to be free to genetically

enhance their children. Nick Bostrom (2005) advocates this position under the transhumanist ideal of individual rights. Yet exercising an option *not* to genetically modify one's offspring is not a right, it is an irresponsibility: "If safe and effective alternatives were available, it would be irresponsible to risk starting someone off in life with the misfortune of congenitally diminished basic capacities or an elevated susceptibility to disease" (Bostrom 2005). Thus, proponents of such techniques acknowledge a technological imperative. Importantly, "diminished basic capacities" is not a neutral term, but one shaped by available technologies and loaded with substantive repercussions regarding the kinds of citizens that society cherishes and the kinds of citizens it judges inferior.

In his own defense of liberal eugenics, Nicholas Agar (2004) notes that parents who choose not to enhance their offspring will be putting their children at a disadvantage, as enhanced children "ratchet up" the prerequisites for being capable of fully participating and succeeding in society. Indeed, they will likely not just ratchet up the requirements, but change them as well. Thus, what is advocated as a freedom or permission becomes instead an obligation that burdens others' "procreative liberties." My decision not to genetically improve my child may leave him unable to succeed in life because of the enhanced competition.

Gregor Wolbring (2008) labels this dynamic "out-ableing" or "the rat race for abilities." In particular, he critiques utopian visions of human enhancements, such as those presented in the National Science Foundation report edited by Mikhail Roco and William Bainbridge (2002). Such visions inevitably extol a certain set of abilities—in this case productivity and a certain form of intelligence. As enhancements for these abilities become available, the unenhanced may likely come to be understood by the enhanced as deficient. More troubling, the unenhanced will likely come to see themselves as deficient as they make their self-image in comparison with widely cherished societal values. Furthermore, society will become structured around the new abilities and the new values, meaning that they will be far from neutral with respect to their impacts on various conceptions of the good.

Indeed, the technological assemblage of material culture always works to provide some with greater advantages than others. The French term for assemblage, *agencement*, gets this point across by signifying that human agency is determined by position within and access to technological systems. Insofar as technology is an extension of the human body, the rich have different—bigger and better-equipped—bodies than the poor. Enhancements threaten to die-cast these differences quite literally into human bodies, perhaps splitting haves and have-nots into, not different classes, but different species.[1]

But the same point can be made through actual, rather than futuristic, scenarios. In 2008, for example, proposed legislation for a U.S. National Neurotechnology Initiative justified itself in part with the incredible claim that 100 million Americans suffer from some form of brain disorder. The bounds of normalcy are clearly being narrowed here under a medicalizing imperative. Initially, stress is considered a disorder, then hyperactivity—there is no logical limitation to considering sadness, shame, or self-discontent as instances of disease and disability to be "fixed" through technological means. In this fashion, what is considered species-typical suffers death by a thousand cuts as the bar of normalcy is continually moved according to a market-driven technological imperative.

Consider the increasing off-label use of "smart pills" such as Adderall by college students in order to boost mental capacity and memory (Garreau 2006). If such drug use is left unregulated, soon many students may feel they have no choice but to pop smart pills just to stay competitive. In a widely reported story from June 2006, eleven cousins had their seemingly healthy stomachs removed because they all shared a gene that signals an increased risk for stomach cancer. Genetic information such as this not only allows for preventative surgery, but makes possible the practice of genetically screening embryos for problem genes prior to implantation. In line with Bostrom's correlate, might we see a time when it is considered irresponsible to procreate without first screening gametes or embryos? Similarly, as regenerative medicine matures—including the ability to grow tissues and organs in the laboratory from patient cells—it will herald changing attitudes toward the human body and societal demand for tailor-made replacement parts. Thus, as technologies expand what we can do, they tend to expand in turn both our obligations and our rights claims.

In sum, the expansion of the private sphere implicitly licensed by instrumentalism's focus on individuals' rights to make "private" decisions creates public quality of life issues (see McGinn 1991). In a profound self-contradiction, the modern image of the self as a rights-holder preceding community has been made radically problematic by the very workings of modern technology in a consumerist society. It is not sufficient to think and talk only about securing the means to acquire the good, because technologies are not mere means—means and ends are inseparable. Thus, the question of the good is necessarily answered both individually and collectively; there is no way to support a non-answer or a neutral point of view. We can only answer it in a more or less conscious or thoughtful way. Rich public bioethics attempts to bring these dimensions into view, whereas instrumentalism pretends that none of this is going on.

Implications for Political Liberalism

Liberal democracies are deeply implicated as regulators and promoters in the development of modern technology. Both liberalism and technology are commonly thought of in neutral terms with respect to human goods. Technologies are neutral means for individuals to use in accomplishing their ends. The liberal state offers a neutral framework that allows a plurality of conceptions of the good to flourish—conceptions that each can choose from both a basic and an ever expanding array of technological means to achieve their ends. The ambiguity noted above is that technology delivers more than it promises. It promises a neutral means to pursue whatever we desire, but in fact develops definite styles of life that are far from neutral. This ambiguity is evident at the outset of modernity, as the early modern founders promised both a neutral arena to pursue the good as one sees it and a definitive vision of the good grounded in a technological mastery of nature.

As Albert Borgmann argues, despite the philosophical foundations of liberal democracy in the idea that the state should refrain from supporting any particular idea of the human good, in practice, "liberal democracy is enacted as technology. It does not leave the question of the good life open but answers it along technological lines" (Borgmann 1984, 92). The opportunities that John Rawls and other liberal theorists want secured in a just manner are conceived of technologically. Access to goods, services, and information require the construction of roadways, health care institutions, media systems, and more. These are not seen as one option among others, but as the basis for having options. Technology is presumed to liberate and enrich us to such an extent that it is accepted as the default condition for the possibility of free choice, rather than a choice among others. In Borgmann's terms, these basic structures are far from neutral in terms of our choice of a commodious or engaged existence, so conceiving of them as basic requirements of justice actually advances a substantive view of the good life.

Of course, implicit in Borgmann's formulation is the monistic assumption that there is one single "technological answer" to the question of the good life. A more realistic appraisal of modern society must acknowledge the diversity of ways of living that can thrive in modern technological cultures. There are still several answers that individuals can give as responses to the material and social conditions in which they find themselves. But the important aspect of Borgmann's remark is that these answers are responding to conditions that are partially created by liberal democratic governments. In regulating and promoting technologies, such governments unavoidably shape the human lifeworld. Their laws (or absence thereof) structure and delimit the range and type of answers that individuals can give to the question of the good life. Governments unavoidably promote some ways of being and discourage others (see Barry 1965). The case for a rich public bioethics is that bioethics institutions can serve as mechanisms for government and its citizens to become more aware of these dynamics.

Yet, following Engelhardt, some may feel uneasy about any association between government and the good. They might concede that a rich bioethics may be desirable, but a rich *public* bioethics is somehow inappropriate for a liberal society. Three types of arguments along this line seem initially plausible.

The first argument is very broad. It contends that because political liberalism is founded on individual liberties, it requires the strong theoretical grounding of the atomistic subject. The self/society divide needs to be true, or else autonomy and liberty would crumble under social determinism. A theoretical debate dominated the literature on liberalism after the publication of Rawls's *A Theory of Justice* (1971). Supporters of

Rawls defended the atomistic subject that is presupposed by the veil of ignorance, while critics pointed out how untrue to life this independent being is. We are in fact, as Charles Taylor (1989) remarks, "dialogically constituted" through our relationships as the self exists only within "webs of interlocution." These webs are constitutive of human agency; to step outside of them is not to achieve freedom but to destroy the possibility of a choosing person at all. Or as Kwame Appiah puts it: "the self whose choices liberalism celebrates is not a presocial thing" (Appiah 2005, 20).

The critics make good points, but without threatening liberalism— indeed they only make clear the conditions within which liberty is valuable. We can define our identities only against a background of things that matter; "to bracket out history, nature, society, the demands of solidarity, everything but what I find in myself, would be to eliminate all candidates for what matters" (Taylor 1991, 40). To value freedom and individuality "just *is* to acknowledge the dependence of the good for each of us on relationships with others. Without these bonds . . . we could not come to be free selves, not least because we could not come to be selves at all" (Appiah 2005, 21).

To imagine a person incapable of constitutive attachments "is not to conceive an ideally free and rational agent, but to imagine a person wholly without character" (Sandel 1982, 179). Our, often unchosen, commitments and attachments are not (only) constraints, but are necessary horizons of meaning and purpose (Frankfurt 2004).[2] Furthermore, though we certainly do author our own lives to some extent, we never simply decide by and for ourselves. My decisions reflect my image of myself, but this image is shaped by my understanding of how others understand me. The self-understanding that motivates my decisions is open to change through interactions with others.

Carl Elliott (2003) makes this point in the context of America's obsession with enhancements from self-help books to Viagra to Botox. Americans in particular tend to convince themselves that "the sovereign individual is in charge." Society is something that gets in the way of personal life projects. But, of course, "society helps make us who we are. America creates Americans" (Elliott 2003, 304). What Elliott diagnoses in America's enthusiastic embrace of enhancements is a bad case of bad faith—unsure of who they are, but certain that they are supposed to be happy, Americans begin to suspect that others have it all figured out. They turn to enhancements to pursue a better life, but it is a better life as defined by the market, or as defined by their sense of what others think is a better life. Thus, what appears on the surface as the individual pursuit of happiness is actually a collective anxiety. Instrumentalism is duped by the surface appearances and thus does not see what Elliott identifies as the ultimate danger, namely, that this collective pursuit of enhancement "may well create profoundly alienated, unhappy Americans who are uncomfortable in their own skins" (Elliott 2003, 304).

The second argument against the public treatment of bioethics is that political liberalism requires the state to be neutral between competing conceptions of the good life; this is a more recent form of the debate between those for and those against the "principle of neutrality." There are two main formulations of this principle (Wall and Klosko 2003). The first is "neutrality of effect," which holds that the state should not do anything that has the effect of promoting any particular conception of the good. I have already addressed this version of the principle. Rawls himself was aware that "the social system shapes the desires and aspirations of its members; it determines in large part the kind of persons they want to be as well as the kind of persons they are" (Rawls 1975, 95). It is just this fact that makes it important for governments to consider arguments for and against possible substantive outcomes of their actions.

The standard response given by defenders of state neutralism is to make a distinction between this stronger version of the principle and a weaker one (see Kymlicka 1989). Following Bruce Ackerman (1980), Charles Larmore (1987), and others, this weaker version of the principle is widely regarded as the most viable and important. It interprets the principle of neutrality as "neutrality of justification." This formulation holds that the state should not justify political decisions with reasons stemming from the intrinsic superiority of a conception of the good. What counts as a "neutral" reason is, of course, debatable and changes over time and across cultures. Nonetheless, the instrumentalist terms of risk, rights, and justice—along with economic growth—are commonly accepted as permissible justificatory speech.

Does this mean, then, that instrumentalism is the only legitimate form of *public* bioethics? No, because the restriction on speech implied by neutrality of justification applies only to that significant but nonetheless narrow slice of politics that involves the making of decisions that are binding on everyone in a pluralist society. Bioethics commissions do not make policy and are thus not bound by the restriction of speech necessary for neutrality of justification.

The restriction of speech for justification means that political decisions about technology (regulation and promotion) will be based on the principles of rights, risks, justice, and economic growth. These neutrally justifiable reasons almost always correlate to the actual intention behind a given technological project promoted by the government. Investments in biomedical technology will be justified according to reasons of health; defense technology spending will be justified according to reasons of safety; transportation and communication technology spending will be justified according to reasons of commerce and convenience.

The problem is that we cannot have only these intended (neutrally justifiable) functions without so-called "side effects." Again, technologies are "forms of life" that necessarily also pattern the human lifeworld in particular ways, but neutrality of justification creates a scenario in which these facts must remain unintended by liberal design, and thus not qualify as part of legitimating political discourse. Technologies will always engender effects far beyond the scope of the neutrally justifiable discourse brought to bear in the formation of political decisions. In effect, we allow public policymakers to consider only a narrow range of outcomes associated with technological change. In light of the unavoidable "unintended" consequences, the broadening of considerations through rich public bioethics is a way to help citizens explicitly consider ethical dimensions that are deemed off limits in justificatory arenas.

The liberal restriction on legitimating discourse is profoundly important. The alternative is to make a controversial moral point prevail through legislation, a strategy that would undermine the virtues liberalism seeks to promote by resorting to force, rather than using persuasion.[3] Furthermore, the principle of the neutrality of justification is meant to avoid government that destroys moral pluralism by coercively imposing a controversial way of life from the substantive principles of a single comprehensive doctrine. This moral domination by the state is what the "leaving-out" of Hobbes and Locke was strategically meant to avoid.

Any "perfectionist" proposal, then, for "putting-in" must also be strategic. As Joseph Raz (1986), Thomas Hurka (1993), and Goerge Sher

(1997) point out, liberal democracies regularly avail themselves of such strategies. Raz especially notes the difference between state neutrality and moral pluralism—the latter can flourish in the absence of the former. He also notes the difference between perfectionist political actions that seek to promote the good and the coercive imposition of a single way of life. Coercion is only one way in which the state may promote the good, and in all but extreme cases it is clearly incompatible with liberalism.

State support for liberal education is a noncoercive way in which the state can use its resources to help citizens choose valuable options and avoid inferior alternatives. A liberal education is not only compatible with moral pluralism; the virtues it fosters—open-mindedness and critical thinking—are required to sustain moral pluralism. Further, since any account of autonomy must include the notion of action with understanding, education is essential for enhanced autonomy through improved judgment and reasoning. Indeed, any truly neutral state would deprive citizens of important goods by not fostering the development of their characters, including their capacities to make sound judgments.

Public bioethics institutions such as the Kass Council are strategic places to explicitly explore a diversity of visions of the good.[4] Like liberal education institutions, bioethics committees should openly and critically assess substantive goods. This is a perfectionist strategy of promoting such goods central to liberal learning as critical inquiry and open-mindedness, but it is perfectionist only in the very modest sense that it is better for citizens to be more fully informed and deeply reflective about the human and moral significance of biomedical science and technology. As public bioethics institutions have no regulatory power, citizens and their elected representatives retain authority to make decisions, including the decision whether even to listen to the advice of such institutions in the first place. This is a far cry from fears that rich public bioethics invites state coercion antagonistic to moral pluralism (e.g., Charo 2007). If implemented well, public bioethics institutions offer an opportunity for the adherents of different moral traditions to refine their positions and expand their imaginations by conversing with those holding other views. Again what seemed a threat to liberalism is in fact an ally.

This introduces the third argument against a rich public bioethics forum, which holds that conceptions of the good are beyond the scope of reason—that there is an asymmetry between what reason can show us about moral obligation and what it can show us about human flourishing. This ethical epistemology draws a strict line in the abstract prior to any particular debate between what is reasonable (the right) and what is unreasonable (the good), and it informed some criticisms of the Kass Council (e.g., Mooney 2001; Norton 2004; Majunder 2005[5]). Insofar as this is a widely held position, it may be one reason for the appeal of instrumentalism and its restriction of moral inquiry to matters of the right. Instrumentalist bioethics here endorses Rawls's distinction between comprehensive doctrines, which are controversial and thus cannot be a legitimate part of politics, and political terms, which retain their meaning without reference to conceptions of the good (Rawls 1993).

But we cannot and do not need to maintain this line between reason and unreason.[6] As we have seen, rights and goods often intermingle, and talk of rights and justice necessarily implies a notion of what constitutes a good society and human flourishing. We saw in chapter 1 that autonomy, a term central to rights talk, points beyond itself to matters of personhood and dignity. Even the supposedly noncontroversial (thus properly "political") notion of harm is informed by substantive worldviews. Thus we see disagreements about what actually constitutes a harm—the despoliation of natural scenery by fields of wind turbines? the publication of a political cartoon that pictures the prophet Muhammad? But even when a harm is agreed upon as such, issues will not always be settled by an appeal to that harm if other principles are held more highly. For example, some object to a ban on human cloning because it would restrict procreative freedom, notwithstanding agreement that the procedure carries a high risk of harm to the resulting child.

Political issues are defined in terms of deeply held values: substantive reasoning intervenes in establishing the conditions for the possibility of politics, even if afterward and on the surface the moral dialogue appears adequately "noncontroversial" (see chapter 7). Moreover, issues and principles once considered controversial and thus not properly political can become noncontroversial and political. Finally, no liberal theorist would suggest that the rights of certain groups of people not be discussed merely because doing so is controversial and implies substantive notions of what it means to be human and to be a just society. Controversy is no reason to stop reasoning.

Mill noted that it is precisely when we disagree with someone on how best to live that we have "good reasons for remonstrating with him, or reasoning with him, or persuading him, or entreating him." Of course, this is not a good reason for "compelling him, or visiting him with any evil" if he chooses differently (*On Liberty* 1859, I). But, again, coercion is only one aspect of politics. Conversing and debating are at least as important. Liberty is largely valuable because it provides the conditions under which we can choose better over worse options through such conversations:

> Liberal conditions — freedom of expression, of association, and so on — are required if people are to be able to find out what is valuable in life. Indeed liberalism's insistence on the freedom to revise one's commitments, to change one's mind, only makes sense . . . if we can be wrong about our goals and can come to see that they can be changed for the better. If they really are arbitrary, why should the liberal accord such importance to our capacity to change them? (Mulhall and Swift 1992, 24)

Claiming that the good is often reasonable is not to claim that considerations of the good should always trump other reasons. It is simply to argue that "in our prior deliberations about which laws and policies to adopt, questions about how it is best to live may never simply be 'taken off the agenda.' In public as well as private life, the operative distinction is not between legitimate and illegitimate reasons, but rather between good and bad ones" (Sher 1997, 5). It is precisely such "prior deliberations" that are the domain of bioethics committees, and it is here that we most require a comprehensive appraisal of the various paths we could take and the ends we could seek in the development and use of biomedical science and technology.

A Rich Approach to Human Cloning

Drawing a line in the sand between private and public or unreasonable and reasonable in advance of any particular case does not protect liberalism. It shuts down conversation, allowing decisions that substantively impact the way we live to be made by default rather than by conscious deliberation. Furthermore, the public-private divide arbitrarily, thus unfairly, includes some voices or reasons (those judged acceptably public) while dismissing others (those judged nonpublic) out of hand. This returns us to Evans's basic normative claim: the public debate about bioethical issues "should not be artificially limited when such limitation favors the interest of one group over others" (Evans 2002, 5). I can now apply these insights to the work of the Kass Council in order to demonstrate its superiority over its instrumentalist predecessors.

In its report *Cloning Human Beings,* President Clinton's National Bioethics Advisory Commission (NBAC) recommended a ban on "cloning-to-produce-children" (NBAC 1997). It did so solely on the basis that somatic cell nuclear transfer (SCNT) was at the time so risky as to outweigh any arguments for procreative liberties. In its conclusion and central reasoning, then, NBAC adopts an instrumentalist approach to human cloning focused on the means to ensure (and balance) safety and rights. It is instrumentalist as well in considering "cloning-to-produce-children" in isolation from other "reprogenetic" issues, including "cloning-for-biomedical-research." But it also calls attention to the limitations, noted above, of a purely instrumentalist approach. Indeed, the NBAC report both calls for a rich public bioethics and takes tentative steps of its own in that direction, foreshadowing the work of the Kass Council.

Members of NBAC were aware that if cloning were safe, then their conclusion would logically permit it. But to leave the matter here would be to stay silent on the intrinsic value (goodness or badness) of what many perceive as a revolutionary technique fraught with cultural, theological, familial, and political implications. This would leave such intuitions unexamined, instead of seeking to critically evaluate why many find cloning-to-produce-children deeply troubling and whether such intuitions are sound or not. This is the difficult ethical work in this case, not determining that a highly risky procedure with a huge failure rate is insufficiently safe. Indeed, as the Kass Council's report *Human Cloning and Human Dignity* notes, "many people who are repelled by or opposed to the prospect of cloning human beings are concerned not simply or primarily because the procedure is unsafe" (Kass Council 2002, 96). Their concern is with a perfected, safe cloning technology and the moral character of the society that would embrace it. The difficult ethical question is whether it is wise to seek to make the technique safe.

Furthermore, the silence of instrumentalism on matters of ends or intrinsic value would be tantamount to deciding the issue by default, rather than consciously with the aid of an advisory body's deliberations. This is significant, because cloning-to-produce-children is not a personal matter. It impacts relations between generations, shapes identities, creates attachments, and establishes responsibilities for care. Given these points, NBAC could not avoid theological and ethical perspectives on the intrinsic value of cloning. The report thus discusses topics such as the proper reach of human dominion over nature and the meaning of procreation and family. And it repeatedly calls for continued deliberation by the federal government and others on substantive issues beyond rights and safety.[7]

These calls raise an important point. Emerging biomedical and behavioral science and technology are themselves driving the need for a rich bioethics. Many of these techniques raise questions about the human condition that go beyond the fair, respectful, and safe treatment of persons (indeed, the meaning of "respectful" and "person" often necessitates deeper thinking). NBAC found itself driven toward these issues despite its instrumentalist tendencies.

As the first federal report on the subject, NBAC's *Cloning Human Beings* assembles in one document an array of perspectives on the intrinsic value of cloning. It elevates a loose-knit conversation to national attention. The result, however, is a cursory and hodgepodge collection of views that lacks systematic development. The chapter on religious perspectives especially comes across as a buffet of voices, giving the impression of incommensurability and irrationality. The report itself stresses the preliminary nature of its discussion and calls for further deliberation. The Kass Council answered this call with its first report, *Human Cloning and Human Dignity: An Ethical Inquiry* (Kass Council 2002).[8] In developing a more systematic, coherent, and comprehensive treatment of the substantive issues, it is an improvement over the NBAC report.

The report opens with a chapter, "On the Meaning of Human Cloning," which sets cloning within broader human and social contexts. The next three chapters provide basic scientific and legislative background. Chapter 5 presents arguments in favor of cloning-to-produce-children and a consensus rebuttal against this technique by the council. Chapter 6 presents a moral case for cloning-for-biomedical-research (delivered in the voice of some council members) and a moral case against this technique (delivered in the voice of other members). Chapter 7 specifies seven policy alternatives, and the final chapter makes and justifies two partially conflicting recommendations, one endorsed by a minority of members and the other endorsed by a majority.[9]

The report illustrates the two main, interrelated facets of rich bioethics, which set it apart from instrumentalism. First, it is substantive because it openly and systematically considers a broader set of ends in addition to the means to ensure autonomy, safety, and justice. Second, the report is holistic in considering human cloning within "its larger human, technological, and ethical contexts, rather than [viewing] it as an isolated technical development" (Kass Council 2002, xxiii).

In chapter 5, the council produces an ethical assessment that is far superior to NBAC's in terms of systematically appraising motivations, intuitions, and principles rather than simply surveying a range of viewpoints. The case for cloning-to-produce-children identifies five purposes or reasons for pursuing the technique as well as three larger moral and political goods—freedom, existence, and well-being—that are often used to defend those reasons. The case against the technique begins with the instrumentalist concerns of safety, consent, and justice. The report credits NBAC and the NAS committee for their work on these issues. It continues, however, by going "beyond the findings of those distinguished bodies in also pointing to the dangers that will *always* be inherent in the very process of trying to make cloning-to-produce-children safer" (Kass Council 2002, 96).

In this rich portion of the ethical analysis, the council critiques the contractual emphasis of instrumentalism:

Not all the important issues can be squeezed into the categories of harms and benefits . . . Important human goods can be traduced, violated, or sacrificed without being registered in anyone's catalogue of harms. The form of bioethical inquiry we are attempting here will make every effort not to truncate the moral meaning of our actions and practices by placing them on the Procrustean bed of utilitarianism.

To be sure, the ethical principles governing human research are highly useful in efforts to protect vulnerable individuals against the misconduct or indifference of the powerful. But a different frame of reference is needed to evaluate the human meaning of innovations that may affect the lives and humanity of everyone, vulnerable or not.[10] (Kass Council 2002, 98)

In constructing this alternative "frame of reference"—that is, a rich bioethics—the council combines both substance and holism in an examination of the human and social dimensions of cloning. This first entails an analysis of procreation and child-rearing, including relations and attitudes between parents and children. As the council notes, it is possible to follow instrumentalism and construe cloning purely in terms of a human choice or "an exercise of freedom" that carries certain risks of physical harm. But this is to miss what is "most unusual, consequential, and . . . morally important," which is the fact that cloning is "a new way of bringing children into the world and a new way of viewing their moral significance" (Kass Council 2002, 99). The report concludes its rich analysis of cloning by reflecting on its implications for identity and individuality (particularly the meaning of origins and genetic endowment for identity), the difference between procreation (begetting) and manufacture (making), the prospects for liberal eugenics, and the implications of all of these considerations for society.

In sum, to analyze human cloning through the lens of the contract-making atomistic self is to miss its fundamental moral significance. It is a technique that alters the procreative and familial relations that are constitutive of the self, underlie our attitudes and understandings of one another, and establish the basis of society. Any adequate ethical appraisal, regardless of its conclusions, needs to take into account these defining moral dimensions of cloning. Yet it is just this rich analysis that instrumentalism precludes. By contrast, the Kass Council report—often by illuminating differences among its members—contributes "to a richer and deeper understanding of what human cloning means, how we should think about it, and what we should do about it" (Kass Council 2002, xxiii).

I conclude this case study by foreshadowing my broader discussion of the policy relevance of rich public bioethics in chapter 7. The cloning case shows that both the substantive and holistic facets of rich bioethics are important ways to improve policy recommendations. As I argued above, only with a clear sense of the goods at stake can policies effectively serve to promote and protect them. Furthermore, a wider context is crucial for comparing different cases to see if different policies are required. For example, in its report the council makes a distinction between cloning and assisted reproduction techniques such as IVF based on the asexual nature of cloning. Holistic assessments encourage such comparative analyses, which can clarify whether techniques or research programs have significant moral differences that warrant different policy actions.

A holistic or contextual approach to cloning has further advantages. Of course, the council report recognizes the prudential value of considering cloning in isolation. Because this is the way it has been treated in U.S. politics, short-term recommendations will need to make sense within that reality. But the report stresses that cloning should also be considered "within a broad context of present and projected techniques that can affect human procreation or alter the genetic makeup of our children" (Kass Council 2002, 97). It is thus important to consider the full range of ethical issues, because they may apply to other areas in reprogenetics. As the report notes, for example, Canada, the U.K., and Germany have crafted their different policies within a comprehensive reprogenetic framework that offers benefits in terms of coordination, oversight, advice, and political legitimacy.

Most importantly, considering research and technology in context is simply more realistic—and therefore more conducive to policymaking—than isolating them. NBAC narrowed its scope to cloning-to-produce-children and recommended a ban. But this is not the whole picture, because policy makers need to know how best to specify and implement a ban. As the council notes, this question is made complex by competing assessments about whether to permit cloning-for-biomedical-research. If policy makers choose to allow this research, then they cannot simply ban SCNT, but must seek alternative strategies, which are explicitly developed in the council's report to a much greater extent than in the NBAC report.

Finally, NBAC sought consensus on an abstract set of principles, especially safety. By contrast, the council chose to develop competing arguments and recommendations. The former approach essentially reduces options, whereas the latter expands them. Part of the role of advisory bodies as public forums is to multiply, assess, and connect options to the relevant goods at stake (see Pielke 2007). In its detailed and manifold policy options and recommendations, the council report far outperforms the NBAC report as a source of policy advice. And this is precisely because of, not despite, its rich approach to bioethical inquiry.

A Rich Approach to Aging and Care for the Aging

In its final report, the Kass Council presents a critique of instrumental thought on the emerging mass geriatric society. *Taking Care: Ethical Caregiving in our Aging Society* (Kass Council 2005b) critiques both the isolationist view of instrumentalism and its limited focus on traditional principles. First, the predominant instrumentalist focus in healthcare on science, technology, and policy "fixes"—as specific means to serve isolated problems—unrealistically portrays aging and dying as problems to be solved, distracting us from the unavoidable need for caregiving. Second, emphasizing autonomy as the primary value is similarly an incomplete response to the reality of interdependence. This reality is made urgent by the effects of science and technology, which extend life but also extend a period of decline during which autonomy is diminished due to enfeeblement, disability, or dementia.[11]

Instrumentalist thought tends to look for instruments, which serve as means to "fix problems." To think about "aging-as-problem" is to resort to the fixes of research, technology, and policy, and there is much good to be done through these means. But as the council notes, this way of thinking is "limited in principle" for two reasons (see Kass Council 2005b, 1–4). First, science and technology are not going to eradicate aging and death. These are not "problems" to be "fixed," but rather conditions to be confronted, either well or poorly, both by the patient and the caregiver.

Second, the traditional policy levers and buttons (budgets, institutions, incentives, regulations, etc.) are of no use without quality caregivers who are not just technically skilled but also equipped with the resources of character to make sound ethical judgments in the numerous, complex situations that they face daily. Successful public policies require virtuous caregivers, but the isolationism of instrumental bioethics advice tends to bracket out the actual practices of care and focus solely on the mechanics of policy levers.[12] What is needed in this context, in addition to traditional policy work, is ethical analysis of what constitutes good care and what it means to age well.

Rather than focus on institutions, then, *Taking Care* addresses caregivers, developing a principle of "best care for the patient now here" and utilizing case studies to hone ethical reflection and judgment. The running motif of this report is that—contrary to the Kantian bent of instrumentalism—there is no procedure to follow in simple means-ends fashion. Rather, quality care requires prudence, "that excellence of heart and mind" that enables one to make wise decisions in variable contexts. Chapters 3 and 4 of the report develop an analysis of this capacity, which can only be done through reflection on goals, goods, and motives in dialectic with attention to the particulars of individual cases.

Examining caregiving and aging not only supplements the limitations of policy and technology "fixes," but also pushes critical thinking beyond the intrinsic limitations of advance directives (e.g., living wills), which are declarations by individuals capable of making informed and voluntary medical decisions. They aim at shaping future care decisions if and when the individual loses the capacity for independent choice. As the report notes, advance directives are attractive to many for their emphasis on autonomy or self-determination and for their promise of a procedural solution to bypass substantive debates about what would constitute best care in particular situations for a particular patient. The free, advance exercise of informed consent would, then, relieve later caregivers of the burden of deciding what to do in the hardest cases. Given this characteristically instrumentalist emphasis on autonomy and procedure, it is not surprising that a previous bioethics committee played a role in the emergence of advance directives in American law and policy (President's Commission 1983).

The council presents two criticisms of advance directives. First, they largely fail to meet their own goals and purposes. Second, the purposes themselves are intrinsically limited.

To make the first point, chapter 2 of the report identifies six shortcomings of advance directives. These include (a) the fact that most people do not have living wills, (b) that those who complete them may not clearly understand their preferences and options, (c) that advance directives often fail to convey treatment preferences clearly, (d) that they often are not transmitted to caregivers, and (e) that even when they are, they often have little impact on caregiving decisions. The council cites a host of studies that call into question the efficacy of advance directives (e.g., Dresser 2003; Fagerlin and Schneider 2004; Burt 2005), some of which draw from the early 1990s longitudinal Study to Understand Prognoses and Preferences for Outcomes and Risks of Treatments (SUPPORT) (Knaus and Lynn 2001). In light of these studies, even strong supporters of advance directives recognize their limitations.

The council concludes that "it is misleading to think that, through wider use of living wills, competent persons will be able to direct their own care simply by leaving detailed instructions in advance" (Kass Council 2005b, 55). This procedural "solution" to the challenges of caregiving is unrealistic, as there is no avoiding an "ethics of care" that consists in a set of practices involving context-specific judgments, which require experience and reflection rooted in character in addition to guiding rules and principles (Tronto 1993).[13] Indeed, a closer look at the empirical realities of caregiving shows that patient autonomy is not just worked out in advance through forms and consultations, but is also realized daily through the practices of care, that is, as long as the caregivers possess the necessary prudence (Struhkamp 2005). The practical reality of care, then, calls for advice pertaining to the character of caregivers in addition to procedures for protecting the prior wishes of patients. The council acknowledges advance directives as "valuable to some degree and in some circumstances" but as a "limited and flawed instrument" for addressing most caregiving decisions (Kass Council 2005b, 214).

The report also critiques the substantive values symbolized by advance directives. In so doing, it identifies the overarching challenge: "Can a society that values self-reliance, personal freedom, and careerism reconcile itself to the realities of dependence, diminished autonomy, and responsibility for others?" (Kass Council 2005b, 4). Personal independence is an important goal, but to emphasize its value just when, as a reality, it is declining, is a mistake: "Living wills make autonomy and self-determination the primary values at a time of life when one is no longer autonomous or self-determining, and when what one needs is loyal and loving care" (Kass Council 2005b, 55).

Furthermore, advance directives can have the ironic effect of undermining autonomy, because it binds the current patient to limitations imposed earlier. The principle of free and informed consent is at best difficult to apply in making decisions so far in advance of the actual situation. It is difficult to see that far ahead and imagine one's preferences. A person's interests can change over time and dramatically so with dementia. Those making treatment decisions in light of new information unavailable at the time the living will was executed, then, must consider what is best for the patient now here, who is a person, not just an inherited set of instructions. Informed consent is important, but it is not a sufficient guide to the perplexities and obligations of ethical caregiving. To consider the well-being of the present patient requires "*substantive* ethical judgments about what being a 'benefit' to those entrusted in our care really means" (Kass Council 2005b, 82).

It is such substantive reflection that instrumentalism eschews and that rich bioethics provides. Chapters 3 and 4 of *Taking Care* are examples of this kind of bioethics.[14] They do not provide answers or make the decisions. Rather, through their detailed, context-sensitive ethical analyses they explore a range of dilemmas and the merits and drawbacks of various responses available to the caregiver. In developing and mixing ethical principles with concrete scenarios, the report enriches the perspectives and widens the capacity for moral imagination and judgment of those who read them. Ethical caregiving is not primarily about following rules, but about exercising a disposition to care. For this reason, successful policies require ethical reflection to "sharpen the gaze and deepen the understanding" of the caregiver (Kass Council 2005b, 149). Thus, a rich analysis of care is an essential complement to traditional instrumentalist policy fixes.

Furthermore, focusing on "fixes" and taking autonomy as the primary value not only detracts attention from developing quality care, it can also deform the experience of aging. The report notes that thinking of "old age as both a bundle of needs and problems demanding solution" creates insatiable desires for more medical cures and breeds discontent with the life cycle itself (Kass Council 2005b, 48). This outlook is most tragic when it leads individuals to believe "that independence is in fact the whole truth about our lives, without giving full regard to those attachments and obligations that bind and complete us" (Kass Council 2005b, 48). Those who forget the realities of our dependence and interdependence are prone to loneliness and bitterness when the illusion of independence can no longer be maintained.

It is better, the council reasons, to explicitly recognize our interdependence by putting greater stock in proxy directives—which designate a decisionmaker—than advance directives of treatment preferences. Proxy directives recognize the value of planning ahead when one can be involved in the process, but they also recognize that ultimately there is no procedural replacement for the substance of wise and caring choices made in particular contexts. Proxy directives not only clarify for medical staff who they should work with in making decisions; being created together with those we rely on, they instruct us in solidarity, strengthening the bonds we share with our loved ones.

Leaving Out and Putting In

The great divide that modernity imagines between self and society has never existed. Humans are, as Aristotle remarked, political animals. Modern technologies only reinforce this basic fact of human existence by weaving tighter interdependencies. Yet at just this moment in history we are witnessing a pervasive individualism that verges on rabid libertarianism, an individualism fueled in part by the fact that modern technology is often designed to give the illusion of independence. One need only think of the experience of driving an SUV to one's single-family home in suburbia—when it comes to experience in the technological age, there is an important gap between reality and appearance (Briggle and Mitcham 2009).

The problem with instrumental thought is that it is confined to the appearances. In its isolationism, it labors under the illusion that humans really are atomistic individuals who can contain personal decisions to a private sphere. This premise supports the conclusion that the only role left for public bioethics inquiry is to secure the procedures and means to support given, individually chosen ends. Of course, as we have seen, that premise is both highly suspect and unnecessary for liberal democracies. This means that there is far more work for public bioethics to do.

The case for a rich public bioethics can be located in the debate within the liberal tradition between, as Appiah labels them, the "Leavers Out" and the "Putters In," or those against and those in favor of drawing "matters of ultimate concern into the universe of political discourse" (Borgmann

1984, 93). In one sense, I have used the Kass Council to advocate on the side of the "Putters In." But our choice is not between leaving out and putting in, because technology precludes the possibility of leaving out, that is, of separating the good from the just and confining the former to the private sphere of individual choice. Our choice, then, is whether and how to make explicit the substance that is always already there and that cannot be avoided with recourse to "neutrality," either technological or liberal. In not thinking and talking about the good, we do not avoid substantive questions. Rather, we answer them—for ourselves and for one another—surreptitiously. We answer them with default activities based on an unthinking obeisance to the routines of our age—routines that are themselves deeply technological, but certainly not for that reason either neutral or unequivocally good.

The kind of rich moral inquiry practiced by the Kass Council offers a way to debate questions that we routinely face but that, with our instrumentalist frame and moral vocabulary, we have largely forgotten how to ask. In a similar critique of instrumentalism, Elliott explained that the price of not retrieving a rich framing of bioethics

> is that by talking exclusively in the language of secular liberalism, we may start to think that way as well; by agreeing that we cannot impose on others our assumptions about meaning and ultimate purpose, we run the risk of failing to think about them at all. The result, if we are not careful, is a moral vocabulary that is altogether flatter: more pragmatic but more mundane, functional but incapable of conveying a sense of deep significance. (Elliott 1999, xxxii–xxxiii)

Over fifty years ago, political commentator Walter Lippmann diagnosed a similar flattening of public discourse resulting from the privatization of ends and purposes. Lippmann recognized the "obvious practical advantage in treating the struggle for the ultimate allegiance of men as not within the sphere of the public interest. It was a way of not having to open the Pandora's box of theological, moral, and ideological issues that divide Western society" (Lippmann 1955, 79). But that Pandora's box has never been closed and as the cases of cloning and the mass geriatric society make clear, biomedical science and technology are opening the box even wider.

FOUR

In Defense of Rich Public Bioethics II

Mind and Body

According to Aristotle, the human is a rational animal. Humanity is simultaneously immanent and transcendent, belonging to and rising above nature. As an integration of reason-passion, the human's rational and moral qualities are continuous with the living world. The human is a complex structure of needs—thus, goods—that often conflict, requiring work to understand their proper ordering. The difficulties of identifying and interpreting human nature sustained ethics for the following two millennia. Descartes, fed up with these endless complexities, cut the Gordian knot. He concluded in the *Meditations* that he himself is simply a thinking thing, and that his body, though attached to his soul, was not part of it but a distinct physical mechanism. This view severed humans from the animal kingdom; animals do not really act, but rather "it is nature that acts in them according to the arrangement of their organs, just as we see how a clock, composed merely of wheels and springs, can reckon the hours" (*Discourse on Method* 1637, 5).

The second great divide, then, is not a split between the individual and society; it is a split within the individual. On one side is the determined, material body and on the other is the self-determining, non-extended intellect. Of course, Darwin reasserted human continuity with the natural world and the animal kingdom, thereby vindicating Aristotle and retying the knot. But the modern reaction to this notion of a clearly hybrid nature has been largely a quest to purify the categories by affirming the dualism of mind-body. Humans are reduced either to bundles of urges (pain and pleasure) or to non-extended, autonomous wills that are choosers and rights bearers. The upshot, in Martha Nussbaum's terms, is a tradition of political liberalism that has long been hiding from humanity by attempting to resolve this inherent tension of spirituality-materiality to one pole or the other. What we need—and the approach that rich public bioethics modestly advances—is to recover a "liberalism without hiding," a political conception of the human being "whose capacities and whose dignity are thoroughly bound up with its animal nature" (Nussbaum 2004, 344).

The mind-body divide is problematic for public bioethics because biomedical science and technology are posing questions about human nature as a whole. In order to protect human subjects from the utilitarian calculations of aggregate pains and pleasures, instrumental bioethics takes to the other side of the dualism. With Descartes and Kant, it locates the human essence in a disembodied intellect. While the Kantian distinction between persons (ends) and things (mere means) is an invaluable moral distinction, humans are not in fact disembodied intellects.

Maurice Merleau-Ponty takes both Descartes and Kant to task on this point. Their "analytic reflection" detaches the subject as a distinct condition for the possibility of human experience. It seeks "an impregnable subjectivity, as yet untouched by being and time" that is the constituting power of the world. But from the very beginning there is no divide between self and world. The human is a being-in-the-world. The body cannot be an object, because it is "that by which there are objects" (Merleau-Ponty 1962, 92). The living body is "the very possibility of contact, not just with others but with oneself—the very possibility of reflection, of thought, of knowledge . . . Far from restricting my access to things and to the world, the body is my very means of entering into relations with all things" (Abram 1996, 45, 47).[1]

Merleau-Ponty demonstrates how dualism and its fiction of the perspectiveless gaze estranges humans from the lifeworld of primordial experience, unlearning the ability to describe the humanly meaningful realm of sight, sound, touch, emotions, and relationships. When we reason practically about what is best to do, we are wondering what is best not in some abstract way, but what is best for the kind of creatures that we are. In isolating a property, namely rationality, as the only feature of moral significance, most Kantian theories stress personhood rather than *human being* and place humans in the same category as robots and intelligent aliens.[2] But our concern in bioethics is with what it means to lead a good *human life* as a whole, as the living, mortal, desire-addled creatures that we actually are. We are not concerned with robots.[3]

Kantian-inspired instrumentalism is mistaken in treating the range and pattern of aims made possible by human biological nature as irrelevant to morality (see Diamond 1991).[4] By contrast, it is from within the lifeworld that rich bioethics takes its bearings. Indeed, the Greek root, *bios,* does not mean animate life (*zoe*), but "a course of life" or "a manner of life" or "a human life as lived," human life as describable in a biography. What are the patterns and structures of this life? What is human life like from *within* this experience? Only from this vantage point can we evaluate the human significance or the goodness or badness of advances in biomedical science and technology.

This dualism of instrumental thought, as with the self-society divide, can sustain only a limited moral vocabulary. Conversation stops just where it needs to begin. There are many biomedical possibilities that could be safe, freely chosen, and fairly distributed, but these properties by themselves leave untouched the most important questions about their intrinsic value—would it be good or bad to pursue them? what kind of lives would they shape and would those lives be better or worse than the ones humans now lead? To answer this question is the wider task of bioethics, and doing so requires an understanding of human nature, because it provides the evaluative standards. In this chapter, I use two sections from the Kass Council report *Beyond Therapy: Biotechnology and the Pursuit of Happiness* (2003a) to demonstrate the benefits of explicitly relating biomedicine to the complex structure of our nature as a whole. This demonstrates how rich bioethics extends critical thinking past the constraints of instrumentalism.

Because this talk of human nature is bound to raise concerns, I will first consider two objections that seek to justify the importance and validity of normative reasoning by an appeal to human nature. The first objection holds that humans are the creatures who "have no nature" and are freely self-determining. But this is an absurd premise and one that is in fact antithetical to freedom. The more serious objection charges that to talk in prescriptive terms about human nature is to commit the naturalistic fallacy of deriving "ought" conclusions from "is" premises. But the objection rests on another untenable divide between "values" and "facts."

We Have a Nature

In continuity with the "blank slate" philosophy of Locke, Jean-Paul Sartre denies that humans have a nature, because this would threaten their freedom: "There is no human nature . . . Man first of all exists, encounters himself, surges up in the world, and defines himself afterwards. If man as the Existentialist sees him is not definable, it is because to begin with he is nothing. He will not be anything until later, and then he will be what he makes himself" (Sartre 1958, 28). Sartre also elaborates a version of Promethean humanism that took shape during the Renaissance. The human falls outside of the vertical, fixed hierarchy conceptualized in the Great Chain of Being. The human is unfinished and capable of becoming anything, especially through its technology. More recently, constructivists have claimed that there is no extra-discursive "human nature." For example, the "cyborg ontology" of Donna Haraway (1991) understands the human not as a particular instance of an antecedent nature, but as a historical construction that is infinitely transformable.

Certainly, we can make no distinction between the "reality" of human nature and its cultural representation that is not itself conceptual, but this does not justify the conclusion that there is no ontological distinction between the ideas we have about human nature and that which the ideas are about (Soper 1995). Indeed, as Mary Midgley notes, "the very idea that anything so complex as a human being could be totally plastic and structureless is unintelligible" (Midgley 1978, 19).[5] Of course to note that we have tendencies (e.g., we are all subject to processes of growth, reproduction, illness, and death) and a preexisting structure is not to submit to determinism. Humans have many "open instincts," which are "programs with a gap" where "parts of the behavior pattern are innately determined, but others are left to be filled in by experience" (Midgley 1978, 53). Humans need culture to complete them, but culture is essential *because of* innate human needs. What we build into our cultures must satisfy our natural pattern of needs and motives.

The nature of a species is what is distinctively common to all of its members. A caterpillar of the species *Danaus plexippus* spins a cocoon and becomes a monarch butterfly. It has certain structural features, powers for performing typical activities, and internal principles of development. The nature of a species comprises "a certain range of powers and tendencies, a repertoire, inherited and forming a fairly firm characteristic pattern, though conditions after birth may vary the details quite a lot" (Midgley 1978, 58). The nature of *Danaus plexippus* is seamlessly descriptive and normative, as it defines what constitutes full flourishing within the pattern of that kind. The criterion for membership is defined not by full flourishing, but by reproduction—being generated from the same *kind*, a notion that admits the immature, the incapacitated, and the aged.

Humans are more multifaceted, complex, and open-ended in their dvelopment than butterflies. So while it is important to avoid monistic thinking that reduces them to *merely* "thinking things," "bundles of perceptions," etc., it is also important to avoid the other extreme in thinking that humans are wholly undetermined bundles of urges, which makes each person entirely a pattern unto him or herself cut from whole cloth. Maslow's hierarchy of needs indicates one commonsense ordering to multifarious needs and goods, but there are many other ways to make the point about a structure to human wants. For example, higher-order volitions are guided by long-term convictions and reasoning. As my first-order volition, I desire to smoke, but I also have a second-order volition, which is my desire to not want to smoke. Others speak of "nested" goods. Not all aims, goals, or preferences make an equal contribution to well-being— I put some off in the short-term to satisfy more important long-term aims. There simply is more to human life than the satisfaction of whatever desires happen to crop up. Some of these desires may be trivial or corrosive when understood within the comprehensive plan of my life. Indeed, the autonomous person requires this hierarchical structure and ordering faculty to identify with her projects as truly her own (see Dworkin 1989).

As another way to put the point, imagine someone admiring a baby and saying, "Ah, that is the good life. All you do is sleep and eat." But upon a moment's reflection, we realize that the good life is not to be had by simply trading in higher and more complex capacities for a simpler set of needs just because they are more easily satisfied. Adult lives that mimic the baby's life would be full of satisfied desires, but these desires would not be satisfying. Those adults would lack goods such as knowledge and autonomy, which are required for formulating a valuable project and sticking to it despite distractions, temptations, and hardships (see Hurka 1993). Again, these points do not diminish the value of those, such as the baby, who do not exhibit the functions of what natural law theorists call "the privileged normal case," because they are members of the human species and of loving human families.

Conservative theorists often uncritically and dogmatically invoke human nature to resist reforms and eternalize class and gender divisions. And indeed the concept of "nature" has long been marshaled by various ideologies to authenticate certain norms, thereby excluding or oppressing various "deviants." The Kass Council was criticized along these lines. It was accused of cloaking a contingent set of norms in the commanding rhetorical garb of nature (e.g., Bostrom 2004; Norton 2004; Nelson 2005; Macklin 2006). Readers must evaluate the soundness of any specific argument presented by the council on their own. This is particularly important given the ease with which "nature" can be used to muddle rather than clarify thinking, thereby supporting irrational and reactionary politics. But I will argue in the next sections that we cannot avoid normative reasoning from human nature, so the question is not whether to do it but how best to do it.

Indeed, a notion of human nature is indispensible for political liberalism. The early modern architects of liberty made human nature their cornerstone, as is signified, for example, in the U.S. Declaration of Independence. As Midgley notes, Rousseau's famous remark, "Man is born free but is everywhere in chains," only makes sense as a description of innate human constitution, something positive and already there, which is in conflict with social deformations. Mill makes the same point: "Human nature is not a machine to be built after a model, and set to do exactly the work prescribed for it, but a tree, which requires to grow and develop itself on all sides, according to the tendency of the inward forces which make it a living thing" (*On Liberty* 1859, III).

Freedom is not an isolated end. It is made valuable by our natural capacities to use our faculties in individual ways. Humans do possess a power to alter their characters, but it is not *only* a matter of their own creativity; they are responding to an underlying nature. A tree does not become a squid. Humans do not invent themselves out of whole cloth. Constraints matter for shaping meaningful parameters of goods and desires that are responded to. Absent these structures, human freedom would not be a meaningful power, but an unintelligible chaos that would in fact more closely resemble a form of slavery to an unpatterned barrage of sensory inputs and inclinations. As the last chapter noted, identity is shaped in response to external elements. Now it becomes clear that it is also shaped in response to internal elements. Self-construction is a creative response to both circumstances and capacities. To say that freedom is in conflict with human nature makes about as much sense, as Midgley puts it, as for the drunk to fight the bed he is lying on. It is not either choice or innate tendencies. It is both.

Finally, the concept of human rights that underpins liberal democracy is founded on a concept of human nature. As MacIntyre noted, "If there is nothing to morality but expressions of will, my morality can only be what my will creates. There can be no place for such fictions as natural rights, utility, the greatest happiness of the greatest number" (1984, 113–14). Modern liberalism maintains that individuals should be free to act as long as they do not hamper the rightful acts of others. But from whence do these binding "should" and "as long as" statements come from if there is nothing but individual will? Either values are nothing more than projections of the will to power, or moral reasoning is informed by standards and purposes not of our own willing.[6]

The Fallacious Naturalistic Fallacy

David Hume argued that desires and beliefs are two distinct phenomena. Beliefs can be true or false in comparison with facts about the world. Desires, by contrast, do not intend to "fit the world" and cannot be tested or falsified. Because beliefs are about the world, and there is only one world, they can be right or wrong. Desires are about us, and there are lots of us, so they cannot be right or wrong in this sense. Factual and evaluative reasoning are two utterly distinct things.[7]

Perhaps no two concepts have wreaked more havoc on common sense than the "objective" and the "subjective" implied by Hume. This distinction forces concepts such as nature (or courage, mercy, injury, importance, danger, or even dirt for that matter) that seem to combine reports of fact with judgments of value into one box or the other. They can be matters of fact *or* value but not both. Yet as Midgley notes, it is only common sense to think "that understanding what we are naturally fit for, capable of, and adapted to will help us to know what is good for us and, therefore, to know what to do" (Midgley 1978, 177). We can "only understand our values if we first grasp the given facts about our wants" (178).

The idea that it is illegitimate to derive "ought" conclusions from "is" premises, then, rests on the assumption that thinking and the world can be made to conform to the clean categories of "value" and "fact." But this assumption is premised on a metaphysics of fact that very few have seriously entertained (see Putnam 2002). The contemporary notion of a fact is the child of modern science, so it is ironic that science—especially since Einstein—and philosophic reflection on science have done the most to overturn the metaphor of the world "as it really is" seen from "the view from nowhere." Reality as we know it, even through science, is not independent of cognition, but is a product of the interaction between humans and the world.

Facts are seldom confined to raw sense data. It is a fact that this is food and that is poison and that therefore this is nourishing and that is dangerous. It is a fact that this thing is the flag of my nation (calling to mind history and pride or shame) and that event is an ancient ritual (calling to mind tradition and reverence). One must grasp standards outside of the physical sciences before one can even "see" these facts: "They are thus never logically isolated from some kind of 'evaluating'" (Midgley 1978, 178). This means that a sociologist aspiring to be value-free must "choose between blindness to the phenomena and value judgments" (Strauss 1953, 52). How, for example, could one analyze the Holocaust without recourse to value-laden words such as "cruelty," or describe an instance of journalistic fraud without terms like "dishonesty" that automatically call forth values? Any attempt to build such a "factual" account would be less true to reality.

So, facts are not so "objective," and neither are values so "subjective" or "irrational," as Hume suggests.[8] This is partly because Hume's claim amounts to absolute cultural relativism and no one can consistently live a life thinking that all values are mere preferences. It also makes no sense because people regularly reason effectively about ethical matters. They do so in society, but also internally. When we want to know if something is good, we direct our attention to our wants. As noted above, these often conflict ("bonum est multiplex"), a situation that calls for some system or scheme of priorities for ordering them. The more free and adaptable a creature is, the more it requires such a scheme. Humans must look to their lives as a whole and ask how that something fits. It is good if it is wanted not just by casual impulse but by the person as a whole on grounds conveyable to others (see Midgley 1978, 182).[9] Reason cannot be simply the slave of the passions, because it must be able to determine which passions to follow. Rather than being an alien, colonial master of the passions, reason grows out of and completes a natural balance of the parts comprising the human whole.

This is the detailed critical thinking entailed in right reasoning from nature. It is what the Kass Council's mission statement refers to as its primary goal of undertaking "fundamental inquiry into the human and moral significance of developments in biomedical and behavioral science and technology." Like any form of argumentation, there are good and bad ways to go about it. One bad way is to make simplistic assertions that "X is (un)natural, therefore bad/good."[10] The good ways involve not just turning to the facts about human nature, but discerning the relevant facts and considering the way they cohere. To discern what is good is a difficult task of distinguishing the good and important from the bad and less important, but it is better than simply deciding the matter by default or through implicit assumptions. The reward will come in the form of identifying the appropriate questions and concerns, expanding moral imagination, and honing arguments that do not just express powerful intuitions or wants, but relate them to human nature as a whole.

Teleology and Modern Science

According to Aristotle, it is the study of natures, as the distinguishing functional features of entities, that both constitutes natural science and provides insight into the *teloi*, purposes, or ends of things. With the moderns,

the scientific understanding of nature came to focus no longer on the natures of different kinds of entities, but on laws (in a very different sense
than natural law, because purely physical and indifferent to any meaningful order of things) that transcend all particulars and kinds.

The modern scientific understanding of nature no longer claims to
answer the question of ends or "what for" for each particular thing. One
may argue that, the points above notwithstanding, modern science prohibits any account of nature as prescriptive. But the expulsion of teleology
was *not* an inductive result of failing to record purposeful behavior in nature. Rather, it was an a priori prohibition—the search for final causes was
suddenly held to be at variance with what it means to be scientific. Teleology contradicts the type of being and causality *presupposed* by modern
science. Its rejection was not the result of science, but rather one of its beginning postulates (Jonas 1966); and it is a postulate that biology, at least,
has had to rethink.

Indeed, Larry Arnhart (1998) shows how teleology is essential to
modern biological explanation. To explain the eye, for example, we need
not just a physiological mechanism, because this by itself says nothing
about the function of the eye. An adequate explanation of the evolution
of the eye requires a teleological account of how optical mechanisms were
adapted for various forms of vision that promote reproductive success:
"The physiological account explains *how* an eye operates. The teleological
account explains *why* it operates as it does" (Arnhart 1998, 244).[11] Darwinian natural science has teleological explanation as its central concern.
Darwin substantiates this point in many personal letters (see Kass 1985).
It is only through such teleological *explanation,* not mere physiological *description,* that Darwinism can refute critics who claim it cannot account
for the rise of complex organisms.

In excluding final causes from external reality (matter), dualism nonetheless saved the truth of the excluded trait in the essence of humans (conscious interiority). This seat of teleology was not disowned, but only sepa-
rated from the external world. Yet this dualism proved untenable in the face
of living organisms, especially humans, which clearly embody and inti-
mately relate the supposedly distinct realms of spirit and matter. Scientific
materialism then inherited a challenge that dualism was able to avoid. As
Jonas explains, "When dualism departs and the *res cogitans* in its organic

foundation becomes itself part and product of unitary nature, Bacon's reference of final causes to the 'nature of man' ceases to have the extrusive effect it had in the dualistic setting; and finally the doctrine of evolution, now inseparable from modern monism, obliterates any vestige of the dividing line on which the whole argument of contrasting 'nature' and 'man' rests" (Jonas 1966, 37). This situation offers two possible resolutions:

> Either to take the presence of purposive inwardness in one part of the physical order, viz., in man, as a valid testimony to the nature of that wider reality that lets it emerge, and to accept what it reveals in itself as part of the general evidence; or to extend the prerogatives of mechanical matter to the very heart of the seemingly heterogeneous class of phenomena and oust teleology even from the "nature of man," whence it had tainted the "nature of the universe"—that is, to alienate man from himself and deny genuineness to the self-experience of life. (Jonas 1966, 37)

The latter option reduces humans to mere matter. Jonas concludes that "through the continuity of mind with organism and of organism with nature, ethics becomes part of the philosophy of nature" (Jonas 1966, 282). Just as dualism is unintelligible so is materialist monism. Neither does justice to the mysterious wholeness of humans and other living organisms.

Nature in Bioethical Discourse

Hume's dichotomy has had the effect of muddling bioethical discourse. For example, some bioethicists (e.g., Holland 2003), concerned to avoid a naturalistic fallacy, define nature as the basic background conditions accepted by a culture. According to this view, the naturalistic fallacy consists in mistakenly labeling certain cultural conventions, albeit very old and entrenched ones, as "natural." Those who denounce some practices as "unnatural" are in reality claiming that those practices will disrupt these cultural background conditions. Such potential disruptions may supply good reasons to prohibit certain technologies. The "natural" here is in reality a psychological coping mechanism—a way to hold on to orienting cultural assumptions challenged by novel technologies. It governs how quickly society can adapt to change, but it is not itself a normative evaluation of change.

But this position slides into the unintelligible thesis that humans have no nature. It also yields a radical cultural relativism. For example, Russell Blackford (2005), in the process of defending this argument, claims that "many background conditions in various societies *should* be threatened ... Some background conditions actually distort cultures and their moral assumptions in highly undesirable ways." He cites the treatment of women as inferior in some cultures as an example (female genital mutilation is one extreme case). Yet Blackford's line of reasoning undermines the conventionalist reinterpretation of nature. By what standards could he justify such a transcultural evaluation? How could he speak of "distortion" absent some guiding image of good or right? He must be appealing to some *natural* (i.e., a-cultural and a-historical) standards. If appeal to a natural standard is disallowed, then there are no objective grounds for challenging the authority of customs or conventions such as oppression of sexual minorities or clitoridectomy. Personal preferences are all that remain.

All reductionists such as Blackford commit this self-contradiction (see Taylor 1989). They dismiss natural standards all the while making judgments that they contend are valid independent of their culture or personal preference. As Kate Soper remarks, unless nature is acknowledged as more than a cultural formation, there can be no convincing grounds for challenging the normative pronouncements of various cultures: "One can only successfully expose those reactionary cultural forces that have been falsely defended as natural from a position that acknowledges the extent to which these are themselves 'unnatural' impositions: cultural dispositions that take too little account of the exactions of natural needs and desires" (Soper 1995, 140).

Soper attacks the extreme anti-essentialism of postmodern sexual theory. She notes that those who deny that there is any "natural" body undermine their grounds for normative criticism of existing practices: "For if there are, indeed, no 'natural' needs, desires, instincts, etc. then it is difficult to see how these can be said to be subject to the 'repressions' or 'distortions' of existing norms, or to be more fully or truly realized within any other order of sexuality" (Soper 1995, 130).[12] Indeed, to reduce the body to a mere cultural construction akin to a watch or any other arti-fact is to paradoxically deny the lived experience and creative self-making that gives constructivist criticisms such force (Soper 1995, 135). Hearken-ing back to Aristotle's distinction between cultivation and construction helps clarify the point: bodies are not entirely biologically determined, but neither are they culturally constructed like telephones or airplanes.

Another damaging effect of the fact-value dichotomy is to force ap-peals to natural standards underground (where they drive debates with-out being made explicit) or shove them into the ill-fitting garb of instru-mentalism. The debates about contraception provide a good example. Some see contraceptives as useful tools for ensuring the safety of sexually active teenagers, while others denounce contraception as licensing im-moral behavior. These different perspectives are based on conflicting phi-losophies. The first sees contraception as a way to have the physical plea-sure of sex without undesired and unintended consequences; the second views sex as a moral act intrinsically connected to procreation. The sec-ond view leads to claims that contraception is unnatural because it dis-torts the proper function of sex.

While it would appear that this is a case where one group is marshal-ing nature as a rhetorical strategy to limit the choices of another group whose position has no recourse to natural standards, if we look more closely we see that *both* sides in the contraception debates make argu-ments about the proper nature of sexual conduct and the moral cultivation of sexual desires for their appropriate expression. A *New York Times* ar-ticle noted that "all parents struggle with how to shield their children from the excesses of popular culture" (Shorto 2006). The article cited a study showing that 95 percent of parents think that schools should encourage teenagers to wait until they are older to have sex. Nearly everyone agrees that there is a difference between beautiful and debased sexual acts (even if they are both freely chosen and safe). In other words, the debate is not at the level of some arguing for a cultivation of proper sexual mores and others arguing for an "anything goes" promiscuity. Both sides at least tac-itly appeal to a vision of the natural, thus, proper expression of sexuality that is more than a subjective preference or cultural convention.

In a defense of liberal eugenics, Nicholas Agar (2004) provides an-other reason why natural standards are unavoidable. Noting the "ratchet" effect discussed in the previous chapter that leads to a curtailment of procreative freedoms, Agar argues for a "moral image" capable of distinguishing between genetic therapies and enhancements. He argues that society should strictly limit the use of genetic therapies to the "prevention of disease" and "maintenance of normal functioning" (Agar 2004, 87). Thus, even some proponents of liberal eugenics ("the freedom of citizens to design other citizens") find the need for some distinction between therapy and enhancement—that is, some standard of what is natural or normal.

Nick Bostrom (2005) is also guilty of this failure to distinguish among cases. He asserts that "it is astonishing that somebody as distinguished as Leon Kass should still in this day and age be tempted to rely on the natural as a guide to what is desirable or normatively right" and that "most thoughtful people" reject "nature as a general criterion of the good."[13] But as I have argued, people regularly appeal to nature, albeit in muddled and surreptitious ways. Bostrom himself is not aware of his self-contradictions in his own implicit appeals to natural standards of normativity. For example, he agrees with Kass that the citizens of *Brave New World* have "stunted" "intellectual, emotional, moral, and spiritual faculties." This implies some standard for nonstunted or normal faculties. This standard could be culturally relative or subjective, which would save his anti-naturalism. But it would do so at the enormous cost of reducing his claims to mere statements of preference.

Indeed, Bostrom's essay is full of his own moral ideals. He favors, for example, a "more inclusive and humane ethics" and believes that health, intellect, talent, and self-control are "blessings that tend to open more life paths than they block." Yet he never justifies these moral goods. If they are to be more than preference or convention, then the implied justification is that these ideals are good for the kinds of creatures that humans are. In other words, humans have a nature that flourishes when faculties are developed in certain ways rather than others and when life paths are opened rather than closed. The question Bostrom poses for any proposed enhancement is whether it indeed would be, in his term, an "improvement" on human nature. The best way to address this question is to critically and explicitly investigate the proposal in light of the whole of human nature, rather than simply assert unexamined ideals about improved capacities and increased control over mental states and moods. In short, the goal is to be critical and careful about what really is an "improvement" or an "enhancement," and this requires fundamental inquiry.

Fundamental Inquiry in *Beyond Therapy*

Rich bioethics elevates this dim, confused moral anthropology to a greater level of self-awareness. This kind of analysis is evident in the discussion of human procreation and parent-child relationships in the council's report on cloning. It is also apparent in the analysis of care and reflection on the lifecycle in its report on aging. One need not agree with any specific arguments made by the council in order to see that "fundamental inquiry" is the kind of thinking necessary for cultivating a greater understanding to guide decisions, both personal and public.

The council's best examples of fundamental inquiry are to be found in *Beyond Therapy*. The report sets out by noting that in addition to addressing cures and relief, the powers of biotechnology to alter the workings of body and mind can be used as well for purposes that go "beyond therapy." Reflecting both the substance and holism of fundamental inquiry, Kass introduces the report: "We have structured our inquiry around the desires and goals of human beings, rather than around the technologies they employ, the better to keep the important ethical questions before us. In a quartet of four central chapters, we consider how pursuing the goals of better children, superior performance, ageless bodies, or happy souls might be aided or hindered, elevated or degraded, by seeking them through a wide variety of technological means" (Kass Council 2003a, xvi).

The report takes its bearings from human nature and seeks a deeper understanding of how various biotechnological possibilities fit within the whole of complex structures of wants and goods. The first question in each scenario is, "What does and will this mean for us—as individuals, as members of American society, and as human beings eager to live well in an age of biotechnology?" (Kass Council 2003a, 23–24). Many techniques seem to offer something good, but which techniques will really make our lives, or our societies, better?

These are questions that the therapy/enhancement distinction will not solve by itself: "relying on the distinction between therapy and enhancement to do the work of moral judgment will not succeed" (Kass Council

2003a,16). Matters of health and normalcy implicit in "therapy" are difficult to define, and the "enhancement" distinction can distract from the important considerations of what counts as a good or a bad use of biotechnology. There may be clear-cut cases at the extremes—taking vitamins
versus implanting microchips in brains—but the interesting questions
are in the gray area. What about laser eye surgery; performance, growth,
memory, and mood enhancers; and preimplantation genetic diagnosis?
There is no bright line between "abnormal" mental illness and "normal"
unhappiness. Judgments will entail investigating specific contexts. Hence
the report does not develop an abstract notion of therapy to stand in for
"the natural." Yet neither does it abandon the standards set forth by human
desires and goods. Contrary to Norton's charge (Kass Council 2003a, 2004),
the council does not view nature as the realm of certainty and "pure and
whole knowledge." Rather, *Beyond Therapy* approaches human nature as
the realm of "pure and whole questioning."[14]

Superior Performance

Humans aspire to improve performance in the activities of life and admire those who demonstrate an excellence that surpasses their own abilities. In this pursuit of excellence, advantages from training, equipment,
and nutrition have long been accepted. Now and increasingly in the future we can also "find help in new technological capacities for directly
improving our bodies and minds—both their native powers and their
activities—capacities provided by drugs, genetic modifications, and sur-
gical procedures (including the implantation of mechanical devices)"
(Kass Council 2003a, 101). In chapter 3, the council asks "What should we
think about obtaining superior performance through the use of such biotechnologies?" (Kass Council 2003a, 102).

Three years after the publication of *Beyond Therapy*, baseball star
Barry Bonds hit his 715th career home run, surpassing the achievement
of Babe Ruth. Far from being heralded as a legendary feat of excellence,
however, Bonds's achievement was widely questioned and condemned.
Some fans held up placards with giant asterisks, signifying that Bonds's
home run total should be discounted or not recorded at all due to his al-

leged use of performance-enhancing drugs. Those placards convey an intuition that some aids to performance legitimately support achievement, whereas others degrade or deform it. What is the nature of public indignation in this and similar cases? Rich bioethics does a better job than instrumentalism in articulating such intuitions.

As the council notes, the "familiar sources of concern" central to instrumentalism illuminate some important issues: fairness and equality, coercion and social pressure, and health risks and safety are all relevant ethical considerations. But the outrage was not in protest that Babe Ruth did not have the same chance to use steroids, nor were the fans with their asterisk signs protesting the risks involved or concerned that Bonds was coerced or duped. The problem is not simply one of inequality, because natural endowments are themselves unequal. Likewise, the problem cannot simply be over coercive pressure, because pressure is inherent to the pursuit of any excellence. And the problem does not concern health hazards per se, because the pursuit of excellence in sports necessarily entails the risk of injury. The council concludes that each of the instrumentalist concerns "has indicated something important; but none gets us to the core issue" (Kass Council 2003a, 140).

Getting to the core requires considering whether the excellence of an activity is affected by the *way* it is pursued. The question is how biotechnological enhancement—though clearly overlapping with training and nutrition—may be different in a relevant sense as a means of achieving excellence. After all, what is meaningful and important about superior performances such as home-run records or spelling-bee championships is not the result or the deed considered in isolation, but who is performing the deed, in what manner, and how the doer and the deed are related. (Think of the difference between today's spelling-bee contestants and those of the future with Oxford English Dictionary chip implants.) "We should not separate the score from the purpose of keeping score in the first place: to honor and promote a given type of human excellence, whose meaning is in the *doing*, not simply in the scored result" (Kass Council 2003a, 143). So, at the core is the character of human agency and what the council calls "the dignity of human activity."

Pitching machines can "outperform" humans, but we do not admire them, because they are not performing as humans. In the human case, "active performance" includes not just the autonomic activity of an organism functioning without conscious choice or direction: rather, "it also includes the self-directed performance of various *chosen* human activities" (Kass Council 2003a, 102). It further includes anxieties, aspirations, and other emotions. Central to the performance is the agent performing and how the agent is related to the activity. The purpose of competitive running, for example, is not to cover a given distance as quickly as possible. Though we have cars and airplanes, we do not for that reason stop running competitively. We still run or play chess even though cars can go faster and computers can "execute" a better game, because these activities retain a dignity unique to themselves as *human* performances.

The home-run slugger on steroids is still a human being, but he is "less obviously *himself* and less obviously *human* than his unaltered counterpart" (Kass Council 2003a,144). He has become more like an animal bred or a machine built for competition than a self-willing, self-directing, human agent. He does the deed (hitting home runs) and he may break the record, but "he is also (or increasingly) the passive recipient of outside agents that are at least partly responsible for his achievements" (Kass Council 2003a, 144). The performance and achievements are less *his*— they are partly attributable to the talent of the pharmacologist who is working with him, and to that degree less the product of his own work. For that reason, his achievements are less excellent. He has not cheated his competitors so much as himself and the dignity of the game. The fans with the asterisk signs are saying that Bonds got his achievement "on the cheap." He was "performing" in the other sense of that term as an illusion or separation of what one does from who one is: "performance as the make-believe acting of actors rather than the self-revealing doings of genuine doers" (Kass Council 2003a, 103). So, what makes an act truly human and truly one's own and how does biotechnology relate to this?

As noted above, human acts entail conscious planning, willing, and choice. The instrumentalist, seeing the human as a disembodied intellect, will argue that there can be nothing more human than a conscious decision to enhance performances through drugs or genetic interventions. This would be precisely the expression of rational will and the human ability "to transcend nature's and our personal limitations in a way no animal can" (Kass Council 2003a, 146).

The report responds to this view by highlighting the mind-body whole of human nature. There is a difference between perfecting a skill by using it knowingly and repeatedly and perfecting a skill by means that bear no relation to its use: "*on the plane of human experience and understanding,* there is a difference between changes in our bodies that proceed through self-direction and those that do not, and between changes that result from our putting our bodies to work and those that result from having our bodies 'worked on' by others or altered directly" (Kass Council 2003a, 129, original emphasis). In training, "*The capacity to be improved is improved by using it; the deed to be perfected is perfected by doing it*" (Kass Council 2003a, 127, original emphasis). The active cultivation of natural gifts is intelligible: "we can understand the connection between effort and improvement, between activity and experience, between work and result" (Kass Council 2003a, 127).

Biotechnological enhancements, by contrast, "make improvements to our performance less intelligible, in the sense of being less connected to our own self-conscious activity and exertion" (Kass Council 2003a, 128). Of course, the home-run champion may still train hard and struggle for the record. But "the changes in his body are decisively (albeit not solely) owed to the pills he has popped or the shots he has taken, interventions whose relation to the changes he undergoes are utterly opaque to his direct human experience" (Kass Council 2003a, 128). He is partly alienated from his own doings. He becomes "better" by no longer fully being himself.

An athelete's decision to take steroids is, in one sense, a rational and autonomous choice. However, "it is a choice to alter oneself by submitting oneself to means that are unintelligible to one's own self-understanding and entirely beyond one's control. In contrast with the choice to adopt a better training regimen, it is a calculating act of will to bypass one's own will and intelligibility altogether" (Kass Council 2003a, 147). The Kantian notion of the autonomous self ironically licenses the erasure of willing by mistakenly supposing it to be unlimited. A given embodiment establishes meaningful parameters within which willing can emerge. Humans can choose to work with and against these limits. But to "choose" to bypass them entirely is not to be a willful human agent, but to be something more like an artifact—a product rather than an experiencing and self-directed person. To remove the limits is not to liberate the self, but it is to nullify one's particular identity that makes the self and self-directedness possible and achievement human and meaningful.[15]

A sprinter is not "a rational agent riding or whipping a separate animal body" (Kass Council 2003a, 147). She is a mind-body gracefully and harmoniously at work, driven by discipline and focus. Further, activity is not generically embodied, but is the work of a particular individual. We all have unique identities displayed in our unique bodies and abilities. In pursuing excellence, we each are cultivating our *own* possibilities. In taking biotechnological enhancements, we are giving ourselves foreign gifts that are not our own. Thus, although it is human to strive to be less imperfect, "it is doubtful . . . that biotechnical transformations of our bodies — or minds — will contribute to our realizing this goal *for ourselves*" (Kass Council 2003a, 149, original emphasis). In other words, we will be someone and something else, neither in full command of our rational will nor in native oneness with our bodies.

The irony of identifying ourselves with pure will or mind is that in freely choosing biotechnological enhancements, "we are choosing to become less than normally the source or the shapers of our own identity" (Kass Council 2003a, 150). Such choices flout the excellence of one's own individual bodily gifts that superior performances are meant to complete and display. Finally, "by using these technological means to transcend the limits of our natures, we are deforming also the character of human desire and aspiration, settling for externally gauged achievements that are less and less the fruits of our own individual striving and cultivated finite gifts" (Kass Council 2003a, 150). The council sums up the argument as follows:

> Biotechnology seems to promise the triumph of the will with less willing effort and bodily excellence in bodies not quite ours: we can become what we desire without being the responsible and embodied agents of our own becoming. A more human course, however, might be accepting that we cannot will ourselves into anything we like, but we can still live with the dignity of being willing, self-directed, embodied, and aspiring persons, not biological artifacts, not thoroughbreds or pitching machines. Better, in other words, to be great human runners with permanent limitations than (non)human artifacts bred to break records. (Kass Council 2003a, 150–51)[16]

Beyond Therapy does not offer answers about which biomedical interventions for the sake of superior performance are or are not consistent with our flourishing as self-directed agents. But it does—far more than instrumentalism—clarify what is at stake and develop a moral vocabulary and set of standards for evaluating different techniques in particular contexts.

Happy Souls

Aristotle begins his *Nicomachean Ethics* with the observation that happiness is the ultimate aim of a human life, sought for itself and never as a means to something else. It is an all-encompassing matter of well-being pertaining to the whole fabric of life. Aristotle remarked that everyone can agree with this much, but on the question of how to define and achieve happiness there is disagreement.

In one sense the point of instrumentalism is to stay out of this debate by seeking procedures that allow individuals to define their own happiness. In other words, instrumentalism intentionally stays silent on this score. But this approach is problematic in a way that Aldous Huxley's *Brave New World* (1932)[17] can make readily apparent. What shall we say about a society where everyone has access, if they choose, to a perfectly safe drug that delivers sheer blissful contentment? Instrumentalism sees nothing ethically troubling here. In fact, lives freely spent on such a drug would suit the image of a disembodied, atomistic will quite well.

But far from being the end of the story, this is just where thinking needs to begin. Would lives centered on such a drug—lives that equate pleasure with the good—be good lives? Most people will sense that the answer is "no." Robert Nozick (1974) designed his thought experiment of "the experience machine" to flesh out this intuition. We want to actually do certain things, not just have the experience of doing them. We want not just to be satisfied, but to have satisfaction as a result of acts, relationships, and lives actively pursued and worthy of satisfaction. Those who plug into the machine or take the drug mistake a lesser substitute (pleasurable mental states) for the real thing. They get a shallow contentment at the cost of amputating their higher and more comprehensive aspirations as well as the actual relationships that give life meaning. This is what Mill had in mind when he remarked that it is better to be Socrates dissatisfied than a fool satisfied. Happiness is not merely pleasure, but entails living well.

My point is not just to defend Nozick. The larger point is that it is better for an advisory body as a public forum to enter the debate and explicitly consider the nature of happiness than to stay silent. Especially now, as advances in psychotropic drugs raise new possibilities for blunting memories and brightening moods, this extended analysis is pertinent to personal and public decision making: Which uses of these drugs are wise? What standards and goods can guide thinking and policy? The technologies themselves drive us to consider the nature of human happiness. Without doing so, we will rely on unexamined intuitions and the inadequate moral vocabulary of risks and rights. In its chapter "Happy Souls," the council once again extends our vision.

The report recognizes that humans have long turned to alcohol and other means to surmount the many obstacles to happiness, including grief, shame, regret, and frustration. But the report notes that recent breakthroughs in drugs to alter memory and mood make possible for the first time a *systematic* and *precise* social pursuit of *long-term* happiness via *direct* biotechnological intervention—a biotech happiness industry. This raises the central question of the chapter: will the "pharmacological management of our mental lives" (Kass Council 2003a, 208) bring us near to or estrange us from true happiness?

Answers will not come in the abstract. In some cases drugs may restore natural ability to find satisfaction in life, working to replace disorder— perhaps caused by crippling despair, unrelenting anxiety, or unrelieved remorse—with coherence and stability. In other cases, however, drugs might offer mere feelings unrelated to actual activities and relationships. Thus, the chapter is replete with contextual analyses of specific therapeutic and nontherapeutic uses of different drugs in various contexts. There is no space here to recapitulate the arguments. I will only indicate the general thrust of the ethical analysis, which provides a fitting way to conclude our investigation of rich bioethics and its perspicacious way of seeing things whole.

Happiness is indeed bound up with human identity, that complex integration of mind-body that the report calls the human soul. What is important here are not just our generic human qualities, "but our particular and unique constellation of them, shaped by our own experiences, aspirations, attachments, achievements, disappointments, and feelings" (Kass Council 2003a, 211). The happiness we seek, we seek for *ourselves*—*I* want to be happy. We would not want happiness if it meant becoming someone else or losing our identity. This implies that happiness relates to memory, which supplies continuity to identity. It also relates to moods—resting atop and informed by temperament or general orientation of feeling—which are expressions of identity, reporting the state of affairs of our world as well as our inner sense of and judgments about our selves.

I limit my focus to the report's analysis of "mood-brighteners." The council uses selective serotonin reuptake inhibitors (SSRIs) such as Prozac, Zolof, and Paxil as a primary example of mood brightening agents, though it occasionally refers to others examples, such as MDMA or the street drug "ecstasy." SSRIs are primarily used to treat major depression and other emotional problems so disabling as to indicate the presence of mental illness. The council considers the ethical implications of the use of SSRIs both for clinically depressed patients and for people whose troubles are not so severe and whose neurochemistry may not be abnormal. Indeed, it considers how the success of SSRIs may be contributing to what seems to be an expansion of the diagnosis "depression" to include lesser and lesser forms of sadness. The council first notes that "new psychotropic drugs create the possibility of severing the link between feelings of happiness and our actions and experiences in the world" (Kass Council 2003a, 207–8). Following Nozick, this matters because we care about the difference between the real and the merely appearing. We care, as the report puts it, about "living truly."

A young man on "ecstasy" may confess his genuinely felt love for a perfect stranger. But his feeling of love is not only incomplete, but also unfounded in reality or knowledge about the woman. The feelings are "neither *true* nor truly *his*"; he is not himself, or "in his right mind" (Kass Council 2003a, 253). The case is more complex with prescription mood-brighteners, because many users profess a profound personality "change" and describe feeling free for the first time to be their real selves or to get into their right minds. For example, the report cites an actual clinical case in which the patient had few pleasures, no lovers or close friends, little to look forward to, and crippling fear and anxiety. After taking Prozac, she became calm, confident, and assertive. She negotiated a promotion at work, where she had been trapped in the same job for eighteen years, and dated several men, eventually marrying one. Such profound changes are not a matter of altering fickle moods, but rather affect underlying identity. The patient's personality is not "changed," perhaps, but rather "enabled." She may not be a new person, but she is newly capable of expressing who she really is. Yet many of the same individuals wonder "whether their newfound happiness is fully *their own*—and in this sense, fully real" (Kass Council 2003a, 255). The concern is especially disquieting for these patients when they come to feel happy for no good reason at all or even when there is much in their lives to feel truly unhappy about.

This raises the next concern that mood-brighteners, insofar as they estrange the emotions from the way life actually is, may prevent responding to experience in a fitting way. It is natural to desire relief from the psychic burdens, for example, of a failed romance or the loss of a loved one. Yet "such psychic relief may also estrange us from the attachments that matter most" (Kass Council 2003a, 257). It is possible to suffer "less than we should," and in doing so we risk "diminishing our appreciation of the depth of our love and of the one whose absence now causes our pain" (Kass Council 2003a, 257). "Nothing hurts only if nothing matters" (Kass Council 2003a, 257). It is foolish to seek to excise those aspects of our being, such as aggression, that seem to cause so much trouble.[18] They are inextricably wrapped up with the goods of life, such as touch and compassion in this case. In the case of suffering, we do not want to remove the capacity to suffer when the circumstances call for it, because it would weaken "our appreciation for the very human attachments that make life most meaningful" (Kass Council 2003a, 257).

More generally stated, though of course it is foolish to actively seek out misery just for the lessons it offers, "life's hardships often make us better" (Kass Council 2003a, 258). A drug that induces a sense of well-being-no-matter-what can undermine the efficacy of (negative and positive) affect, resulting in "a life in which fitting feeling can no longer guide or spur us toward living well" (Kass Council 2003a, 260). The citizens of Huxley's dystopia have lost the capacity for yearning. They are content and thus never pursue a life "with the ups and downs that come from having aspirations self-consciously chosen and ardently pursued" (Kass Council 2003a, 260).

A broader concern is the "medicalization of self-understanding," or viewing ordinary affective life through the lens of mental disorders. A person who attributes sadness or discontent to sickness may be spared the difficulty of changing the way he lives. He can take mood-brighteners without a guilty sense that something is missing. But there is a cost to this apparent benefit, because "one reconceives sadness as sickness only by emptying it of psychic or spiritual significance and turning it into a mere thing of the body" (Kass Council 2003a, 261). If happiness is a matter of neurotransmitters, it can no longer be seen as "a spiritual achievement or the fruit of a life well lived" (Kass Council 2003a, 261). Of course it is appropriate to medicalize conditions that are illnesses, but society risks diminishing the very purposes and attachments that drive meaningful human lives if it treats every troubled state of the soul as an illness.

Thus, it is important to distinguish uses that return people to a functioning whole responding appropriately to reality (therapy) from those that do not. Common concerns about safety point to something deeper, past the "clear and present danger" of physical harm, to the wider threat of medicalizing the human soul.

Again, the benefits of extending critical thinking lie in identifying the relevant questions and the goods at stake and developing a moral vocabulary for assessing specific cases. In the conclusion to this chapter, the council also formulates a general guiding principle to aid decisions about the appropriate use of mood-brighteners. The goal is to achieve mental health, which can be understood in light of the above analysis as feeling rightly or appropriately. Doctors should use mood-brighteners when they can help patients "achieve an appropriate relationship between their circumstances, inner life, and possibilities for action, so that they are able to feel joy at joyous events and sadness at sad ones, to marvel at the world's wonders, resist cruelties, and all the while strive to develop their talents, honor their obligations, and cherish their friendships and loves" (Kass Council 2003a, 265–66). A well-balanced, integral—that is, healthy—life that resonates in tune with the world is the goal, not a life of untroubled ease divorced from reality.

Seen from an instrumentalist perspective, the moral and political intent of modern liberalism is to create the "universal and homogenous state," in which all people are respected as free and equal. Matters of truth, reality, and meaningfulness can be set aside as simply the products of each individual's freedom to express opinions. This is the instrumentalist sovereignty of freedom. Yet, we have seen the inadequacy of this picture of human beings. Humans are interdependent, embodied creatures. In the conclusion of *Beyond Therapy*, the council argues that the ultimate danger of a pervasive instrumentalism is that we will come to see the human solely in "material or mechanistic or medical terms" and not in "psychic and moral and spiritual ones" (Kass Council 2003a, 308).[19] We need to see the human as a "creature 'in-between,' neither god nor beast, neither dumb body nor disembodied soul, but as a puzzling, upward-pointing unity of psyche and soma whose precise limitations are the source of its—our—loftiest aspirations, whose weaknesses are the source of its—our—keenest attachments, and whose natural gifts may be, if we do not squander or destroy them, exactly what we need to flourish and perfect ourselves—as *human* beings" (Kass Council 2003a, 308).

PART II

The Politics and Policy
of Public Bioethics

FIVE

The Kass Council
as Institution and Lightning Rod

Substance and holism comprise the essence of rich bioethics as an ideal and set it apart from the formalism and
isolationism of instrumentalist bioethics and the wider instrumentalist habit of mind that is a legacy of our modern
inheritance. Part I demonstrated the superiority of a rich
approach to public bioethics. Yet if we adopt a holistic mindset of our own, we quickly see that public bioethics is more
than ideas and arguments distilled from reports. These ideas
and arguments are inseparable from the political realities
that generate them. Any rich public bioethics must take institutional form, thus introducing the need to judge the appropriateness and success of the institution according to
the criteria of its procedures and conduct. Indeed, one of
the central lessons of the Kass Council is that good ideas
are not enough to accomplish the goals of improved understanding and action.

Thus it is crucial to consider how rich public bioethics
is practiced and perceived. In part II, then, we will turn toward the political and institutional realities of doing rich
public bioethics, shifting focus from the arguments to the
processes that led to the reports, the public perception of
those processes, and the implications of the processes for

politics and public policy. The ideas of rich bioethics both continue and transcend the ideas of instrumentalism. Similarly, many processes of public bioethics remain unchanged whether its approach is formal or substantive, isolationist or holistic, and public perception of those processes may also be quite similar—after all, the Kass Council was certainly not the first bioethics commission to stir controversy. Nonetheless, as the Kass Council demonstrated, certain choices regarding membership, mission, and procedures will be more conducive to a rich public bioethics, and these choices along with the ideas and arguments they yield generate a commensurate amount of increased scrutiny from professional bioethicists, scientists, and other members of the public. Evans is right to warn that "we should be very cautious" about a bioethics advisory committee orchestrating a deliberation over ends (Evans 2002, 201).

This chapter will show how rich public bioethics was practiced by the Kass Council and how its practices were perceived by certain audiences, especially bioethicists and scientists, who were largely successful in sullying the council's public image as it became a lightning rod for conflicting cultural, professional, and political perspectives. I will focus attention on those aspects that were especially conducive to, or even necessary for, a *rich* bioethics commission—its membership and its procedures. I will then survey the two main public criticisms faced by the council: that it was politicized and that it was irrelevant. These criticisms can and have been made against instrumentalist public bioethics, but in the case of the Kass Council they were often related to its mandate to conduct a rich bioethics. Many charges of politicization maintained that—contrary to my argument in part I—rich inquiry was no more than partisan "bioconservatism," and many complaints about policy irrelevance stemmed directly from the deeply reflective mode of inquiry native to rich bioethics. In the following two chapters, I take up these criticisms in turn and offer my own evaluations.

Membership

The membership of advisory committees is one of their most important elements, as the kind of work that gets done, its public reception, legitimacy, and success, depend to a large extent on the people involved and on how they were selected (see Jasanoff 1990; Hilgartner 2000). A council committed to rich public bioethics will clearly require a membership that is both able and willing to think substantively and holistically. Its success will depend on an openness to and skillfulness in a certain *way* of thinking, which is contrary to much of modern analytic ethics and thin accounts of liberalism. But it does not require a partisan or ideological commitment to any particular conclusions or methods. Many types of substantive arguments are put forward about human meaning and living well within the context of the rich bioethics approach. They can range from technological optimism to pessimism. Indeed, as Evans (2002) argued, the problem with the thinning of public bioethics is that a substantive conversation held in the open between deeply divergent perspectives was driven underground or forced into the inadequate moral lens of instrumentalism.

The membership of the Kass Council makes sense when seen in light of the goal to revive this substantive conversation. This is especially true of Kass himself, who had over the years developed a systematic critique of instrumental conceptions of the human condition. He also developed his own rich alternative, which he often called a "richer bioethics" (see Kass 1971; 1985; 2002; Kass and Wilson 1998).[1] Along the way, Kass was labeled by many scientists and bioethicists as a bioconservative, a label that seeks to reduce his philosophical position to partisan politics, and his appointment as chair by President Bush immediately raised suspicions of partisan stacking. But the charge of bioconservatism greatly misrepresents the nature and underestimates the profundity of Kass's philosophical position within the constellation of reflection that has come to be known as "bioethics" (see Vogel 2006).

Although he does often espouse positions associated with cultural conservatism (e.g., Kass 1979; 1991; 1997), Kass's thinking is neither reductive nor partisan. His complex and nuanced approach does not proffer any simplistic, universal conclusions about banning technology or forbidding science. Drawing from philosophical conversations spanning Aristotle through Leo Strauss and Hans Jonas, Kass has developed a radical critique of modernity, especially modern natural science and subjectivist, instrumentalist versions of political liberalism. Lawrence Vogel (2006) argues that Kass's position is best understood as "natural law Judaism." One important theme is his general skepticism about an overextended technological attitude, a standpoint that aligns him with many of the ancient thinkers and sets him in sharp contrast to modern economic conservatism with its often self-contradictory embrace of technological innovation. Rather than engage Kass on the subtleties of this theme or his "natural law Judaism" more broadly, however, many critics have preferred to invent and attack a straw man version of Kass (e.g., Wright 2001; Bostrom 2005; Charo 2007).

Kass, whose degrees are in medicine and science, worked originally as a researcher at NIH, but in 1967 his interests shifted from doing science to thinking about its human meaning. In that year he wrote a letter to the editor of the *Washington Post* regarding the cloning of tadpoles and what he considered to be the cavalier attitude of biologist Joshua Lederberg about the profundity of the issues that cloning raised. Kass has since become an unusual interdisciplinarian, having his training in the biological sciences but the majority of his publications in the humanities. He began writing on the ethical implications of biomedicine, working with many founders of the field of bioethics and served on the Committee on the Life Sciences and Social Policy (1970–1972) of the National Academy of Sciences.[2] Kass held teaching positions at St. John's College, the Kennedy Institute of Ethics at Georgetown University, and the University of Chicago, where he became acquainted with Leo Strauss. During his time as council chair, he served as a professor at the University of Chicago and a fellow at the American Enterprise Institute.

Some critics of Kass's philosophical views testify to his open-mindedness in exploring points of disagreement (Galston 2001). This kind of open disagreement on substantive points and the virtues required to disagree in a civil and productive manner are essential to rich bioethics. In orchestrating reports that, as I have argued, successfully broaden moral imagination and deepen understanding, Kass proved a capable leader of a rich moral conversation. Unfortunately, the vast majority of Kass's critics shirked this debate by simply dismissing him, and by extension the council, out of hand as a mere partisan cog.

As we will see, much was made of whether the membership of the Kass Council was sufficiently diverse. Of course, diversity can refer to professions or expertise,[3] gender, political views, or a number of other variables. Most important for my thesis is the lack of diversity that is necessary to maintain instrumentalist bioethics. The members of such committees may be diverse in certain ways, but the shared assumption is that a language of risks and rights is the most appropriate approach both for assessing the issues and for demarcating the bounds of conversation appropriate to a federal entity. As an ideal, rich bioethics is more diverse in its approach because it requires explicitly assessing the merits of substantive opposing views. It requires reviving the kind of rich conversation that Evans identified in the debates of the 1960s.

Though greater care could have been taken to create a balanced representation of perspectives in both membership and staff, the Kass Council did approximate the ideal of substantive diversity, as became apparent from the differences that emerged among members with opposed ethical and policy commitments. The best example of this kind of disagreement was the split on cloning-for-biomedical-research, where members' commitments stemmed demonstrably from various sources, including different religious traditions, natural law theory, communitarianism, and scientific-secular-liberal humanism (see also Ferguson 2002).

First, religion played some role in the outlook of many members, including Kass, who is deeply influenced by Judaism (e.g., Kass 2003). Three members in particular approached bioethics principally from theological grounds. Mary Ann Glendon, a renowned international and constitutional lawyer who was appointed U.S. ambassador to the Holy See, drew from Catholicism in both defending human rights and critiquing the overemphasis on individualism and "rights talk" in U.S. political discourse (1991).[4] William May (2008), a founding fellow of the Hastings Center and a member of the Clinton Task Force on National Health Care Reform, represented another perspective rooted in Catholicism. Gilbert Meilaender (1995), a professor of Christian ethics influenced by Paul Ramsey and C. S. Lewis, advanced his own critique of instrumentalist bioethics.

Second, though often drawing from theology, Robert George (1993; 1999) and Alfonso Gómez-Lobo (2002) primarily defended a natural law ethics. They were in this sense allied with Kass as well as with Peter Lawler (2002) and Paul McHugh (2006), who developed similar critiques of the impoverished, instrumentalist modern moral vocabulary and its flattened image of humanity. Francis Fukuyama similarly espoused an Aristotelian natural law perspective, particularly in the fundamental claim that notions of right and wrong are ultimately based on human nature (see Fukuyama 2002, 12). Michael Sandel (1982) is one of the leading communitarian critics of contractarian theories of human social life, which grounded his own defense of the "giftedness" of life and his critique of instrumental bioethics (Sandel 2004; 2007).

A third core group of council members were boosters of scientific research and defenders of individual autonomy, whose presence highlights the importance for rich bioethics of including instrumentalist perspectives. This group included the three natural scientists on the council — Janet Rowley, Michael Gazzaniga, and Elizabeth Blackburn — as well as the physician Daniel Foster.

Rowley, an internationally renowned cell biologist and geneticist, implicitly accused the council of being captured by the "conservative right" in her personal statement in *Taking Care* (Kass Council 2005b, 229–30). There she argued for the compassion inherent in respecting individual rights such as those expressed in advance directives. Gazzaniga (2004; 2005; 2006), a neuroscientist, was perhaps the most radical pro-science member, often flatly disagreeing with Kass. For example, in his personal statement in *Reproduction and Responsibility,* Gazzaniga referred to the human embryo as a "miniscule ball of cells in a Petri dish" (Kass Council 2004b, 238).[5] Blackburn, a highly regarded cell biologist, also favored stem cell research and focused her remarks in council meetings on the efficacy, safety, and integrity of the science. Foster, a professor of internal medicine and intermediary metabolism specializing in diabetes research, expressed a very similar perspective throughout council meetings.

Finally, it is important to recognize the crucial role played by the staff of a bioethics committee, who prepare working papers and draft reports, facilitate communication, and handle other aspects of transitioning from meetings to final reports. As just one example, the staff authored a 132-page discussion document that served as a diagnostic overview of regulatory and oversight activities relating to reproductive technologies, and helped inform the creation of *Reproduction and Responsibility.* The staff wielded a significant degree of power in shaping the reports, which served as the official voice of the council.

The council staff was headed by an executive director, Dean Clancy; he was followed in the position by Richard Roblin, who was appointed by the Secretary of Health and Human Services in consultation with Kass. Many members of council staff, including Eric Cohen (2004; 2006), Yuval Levin (2000; 2003), Peter Berkowitz (1999; 2003), and Adam Wolfson (2000; 2003), were affiliated with conservative-leaning publications. This naturally led to suspicions of inappropriate backstage partisanship, as we shall see below.

Procedures

Bioethicist R. Alta Charo argued that the Kass Council was different from previous bioethics commissions, but not because it practiced a rich bio-ethics. Rather, in her view, the council was politicized to an unprecedented degree: it incorporated politics into its work "with a concerted effort to promote a particular political philosophy, and pursue[d] this philosophy through its membership and its staffing" (Charo 2004, 308). She went on to contend that because many council members and staff were affiliated with conservative political groups and publications, the council practiced nothing more than neoconservative, dystopian bioethics. As we will see, many others shared this view.

In part I, I argued at length that the council's work represented a new kind of bioethical inquiry and was thus far more than a continuation of petty partisanship. On this view, Charo is wrong to suggest that previous, instrumentalist commissions "were generally free of ideology" (Charo 2004, 310), at least if she means by this that they were somehow philo-sophically "neutral." Instrumentalism frames moral inquiry and our moral image of humanity in a determinate way that is far from neutral.

Nonetheless, as I will argue in the following chapter, Charo and oth-ers were rightfully suspicious of inappropriate politicization in the se-lection of members and staff. When the fact of conservative affiliations is coupled with the nontransparent nature of the selection process, it is only reasonable to expect suspicion and resistance from groups that rightly feel underrepresented. This leads us to another important point: that the procedures employed by bioethics committees shape their operation, the way they are perceived by the public, and thus their final success in providing advice, deliberation, and education. Certain procedural choices are necessary to fostering a rich public bioethics. These procedures pertain both to the initial structuring of bioethics committees within legislative and institutional frameworks and to the operation of the committees themselves as they interpret and translate broad mandates into specific actions.

I have already mentioned the importance of transparency and balance in member selection, both of which were made problematic in the case of the Kass Council because President Bush retained sole authority for appointing and dismissing council members and for naming the chair. Transparency and inclusiveness are similarly important considerations in the creation of the mission statement. This aspect of the council's formation was also draped in secrecy, which added to the kind of suspicion voiced by Charo. The mission statement is obviously crucial to fostering or inhibiting a rich kind of bioethical inquiry. The Kass Council's mission called on it to undertake "fundamental inquiry," which, as we saw, is a shorthand way of expressing rich bioethics. A broader administrative consideration deals with the institutional home of bioethics committees. The Kass Council—like previous commissions—was housed within the executive branch, which is yet another way in which actual and perceived politicization can infect public bioethics. A mandate to perform fundamental inquiry is obviously essential to rich public bioethics, but the chances of success are hindered if this mandate is not operationalized and institutionalized in ways that are perceived as legitimate (see chapter 6).

Procedures regarding meetings are important for determining their level of openness, the type and amount of public participation, and their location. NBAC and some other previous committees traveled throughout the country, which can be an effective mechanism for sparking public interest and bolstering legitimacy. The Kass Council, however, held every meeting in the Washington, D.C., area, which contributed to a "cloistered" image, even though council meetings were by law open to the public and included time at the end for public comment.[6] All transcripts, along with working papers, reports, and other documents, were made available on its Web site.

Some of the most important procedures pertain to the transition from meetings to official reports. Once again, transparency and inclusiveness are valuable in the process of translating the backstage discussions into the formal reports that serve as the primary public voice of committees as a whole. The council was unusual in not needing to seek consensus on the issues, although consensus could and did emerge on certain issues (see Moreno 1995). But the council did require consensus over how dissent was to be expressed in its reports. It was important that the entire committee be able to own the final report, which entailed finding ways to manage dissent that were acceptable to all the members. The Kass Council employed a variety of mechanisms for conveying dissent, including personal statements, competing recommendations, and footnotes.

Finally, the council had flexibility in its procedures for selecting topics. Indeed, it may have had flexibility to a fault, as topic selection procedures—though guided by some general criteria, including urgency, the need for policy guidance, connection to federal science policy, and the existence of other entities capable of addressing the topic—were extremely informal. As Kass said in the January 16, 2004, meeting, the process is to "invite some people in, have some discussions amongst ourselves, land on a topic that is appropriate." This informality may have contributed to some criticisms that the council did not address the most pertinent bioethical topics. But the council's choice of issues stemmed also from the fact that a rich approach is more relevant to certain topics than to others. For example, because access to health care is primarily a question of distributive justice, in addressing this issue a rich bioethics approach would probably play a subordinate role, giving way to more traditional instrumentalist principles. Once again here we see that rich public bioethics is intended as a way to complement, not replace, other models of public bioethics.

Controversies and Criticisms

The Kass Council became a lightning rod for public debate within the polarized context of American politics and the divisiveness of morally charged bioethical issues. It was subject to multiple interpretations regarding its successes and failures. The council drew heavy fire from bioethicists, scientists, transhumanists, and even some council members, while a smaller group of scholars, primarily represented in conservative publications, came to the council's defense.

In part I, I addressed criticisms that the council's rich public bio-ethics inappropriately and irrationally advocated a substantive vision of the good life. There were, however, two other, often related, criticisms of the Kass Council. First, the vast majority of criticisms centered on the charge that the council was politically co-opted by the conservative right and thus not a forum for independent ethical analysis. Second, many argued that its contemplative style and emphasis on what one reviewer called the "sexy" issues in bioethics divorced it from pressing matters of policy. In each case, defenders of the council, including some council members, offered contrary evaluations. This clash of assessments is rooted in arguments that can be evaluated by norms of reasoning grounded in the evidence of the council's work. I will provide my own assessment of the charges of politicization and irrelevance in chapters 6 and 7, respectively.

Politicization

Fletcher and Miller labeled the gravest peril of public bioethics "political co-optation" or "political capture," which "distorts ethical reflection by imposing partisan political demands or constraints" (Fletcher and Miller 1996, 157).[7] They argued that public bioethics should enable decision makers to take advantage of diverse, balanced ethical reflection insulated from partisanship and the pressures of interest-group politics.[8]

Of course debates about politicization in the federal advisory process are not new (Primack and von Hippel 1974; Jasanoff 1990), but a confluence of events served to make the Kass Council exceptionally electric. The contentious 2000 presidential election left many denying the legitimacy of Bush's presidency. This heightened the level of scrutiny on the process of creating the council, as well as on the council's actions. The morally charged nature of current biomedical issues including embryonic stem cell research and the Terri Schiavo affair (2004–2005) further heightened emotions and raised the political stakes. Finally, the "culture wars" were revitalized during the Bush administration, especially in terms of secular/religious divides on issues such as the teaching of evolution. Thus it was a momentous understatement when Larry Arnhart noted that the members of the council engaged in conversation "about the deeply controversial moral issues provoked by modern science and technology in a political arena of partisan conflict and moral diversity" (Arnhart 2005, 1482). The council did not have the luxury of working within a social context of solidarity.

During the Kass Council's existence, numerous accusations arose that the Bush administration politicized science and the federal advisory system. Indeed, shortly before Kass stepped down as chair, science journalist Chris Mooney released his book *The Republican War on Science* (2005), which both reflected and fueled widespread perceptions that the Bush administration solicited and listened only to the advice it wanted to hear. Several groups raised concerns about bias and conflicts of interest among the roughly 950 U.S. federal advisory bodies. For example, in 2003 a report by the Union of Concerned Scientists (UCS) on the politicization of science directly accused the Kass Council of misusing science to uphold a preestablished political agenda (Union of Concerned Scientists 2004). In 2004 the National Academies Committee on Science, Engineering, and Public Policy (COSEPUP) released a report entitled "Science and Technology in the National Interest: Ensuring the Best Presidential and Federal Advisory Committee Science and Technology Appointments."[9] The report issued recommendations for revising the appointments process in light of continuing allegations of politicization. Another report put out by the Federation of American Scientists (2004) took up similar issues in hopes of strengthening the federal advisory process. Still another response to these developments was a 2004 report issued by the U.S. General Accounting Office (GAO) entitled "Federal Advisory Committees: Additional Guidance Could Help Agencies Better Ensure Independence and Balance" (USGAO 2004).

Complaints rang out from the very beginning, with the formation of the council and Bush's selection of Kass as its chair (e.g., Mooney 2001). The process of naming members and authoring the mission were viewed by many as nontransparent—a means to exclude a full range of voices in shaping the council's membership and mission. For example, bioethicist Arthur Caplan (2002) argued that the council was stacked with political conservatives who would not challenge President Bush's values or policy positions. Bioethicists George Annas and Sherman Elias (2004) claimed that the council was "neoconservative" and "made public bioethics the servant of politics."[10] Charo argued that the council was "suspicious of technological advance" and "opposed to . . . moral pluralism." Further-more, she contended that the council was "a tightknit circle of conservative and neo-conservative figures on what was heralded as a balanced council designed to reflect the range of opinions in the public and capable of considering all points of view. Instead, it more strongly resembles organizations with an openly partisan agenda" (Charo 2004, 310). Lawrence Vogel (2006) argued that the Bush administration saw Kass as its "official standard-bearer" for a neoconservative bioethics agenda. Numerous similar accusations were made (e.g., Gillespie 2002; Weiss 2002; Anderson 2004; Manjoo 2004; Meslin 2004).

The council itself was divided on this point. In the final meeting Robert George stressed "the remarkable diversity of points of view on the Council."[11] Kass (2005) and several others concurred with George on this point, often citing the difficulty the council had in coming to agreement on certain points, while council staffers Cohen (2006) and Berkowitz (2002) argued that the council was more ideologically diverse than previous bioethics committees. However, Blackburn and Rowley argued that the council represented the "political distortion of biomedical science," rather than a "full range of bioethical views" (Blackburn 2004a; Blackburn 2004b; Blackburn and Rowley 2004; Blackburn 2005).

Timothy Noah (2004) traced the partisan bias of the council back to the July 9, 2001, meeting between Bush, bioethicist Daniel Callahan, and Kass. Noah argued that Kass invited Callahan in the full knowledge that they shared similar views about embryonic stem cell research. Noah claimed that this move established a pattern by both Bush and Kass of pretending to seek out representative, balanced debate while in fact perpetuating only a one-sided ideological inquiry.

Other observers, though not as numerous, defended the council's diversity of views. Their claims are given empirical grounding in the fact that the council retained deep divisions on moral questions. Indeed, permanent dissent often remained and is noted in many of the reports. The split decision on cloning-for-biomedical-research is one data point suggesting differences of views on the council.[12] Some saw the council as politically balanced and serving as a gadfly to both liberals and conservatives. Bioethicist Carl Elliott (2004) took this stance on *Beyond Therapy*, claiming that it was "ideologically balanced." Still others defended the ability of Kass to lead a balanced and fair-minded inquiry into bioethical issues. Conservative historian Gertrude Himmelfarb called Kass "wonderfully open-minded" (in Wilkie 2002). Callahan asserted that, although Kass has strong views, "people who totally disagree with him find him a wonderful person to dialogue with" (in Wilkie 2002).

In a personal interview, council member Rebecca Dresser identified herself as a liberal bioethicist who in general disagrees with Kass's philosophical and policy positions (Dresser 2005). But she emphasized that Kass is open to arguments with anyone and does not shut conversation down. She noted that a look at the transcripts should convince skeptics that some members constantly disagreed with Kass and that he encouraged this. In a personal interview, Gazzaniga insisted that Kass always invited dissent and encouraged all members to articulate their ideas and questions. He felt that Kass was never heavy-handed in leading council discussions. In fact, Gazzaniga remarked that Kass sometimes helped him to improve his positions even if they differed from those held by Kass (Gazzaniga 2006b).

Others have made similar remarks about Kass (Wilkie 2002; Holden 2004). For example, *Science* writer Stephen Hall (2002) wrote about the deliberations leading to the council's cloning report:

A funny thing happened to this "stacked" council on its way to a supposedly foregone conclusion. The intellectual arguments were spirited and profound and, in public at least, the stridency of Kass's written views did not influence his public stewardship of the conversation. He proved to be a nimble and fair-minded moderator, giving all points of view their due and egging on all participants to better articulate and defend their position.[13] From the beginning, he acknowledged that the council was unlikely to reach a consensus but insisted that the group produce a document that, as he put it, "everyone can own."

Similarly, bioethicist Kathy Hudson, director of the Genetics and Public Policy Center at Johns Hopkins, wrote about *Reproduction and Responsibility*:

The scope of the document's inquiry has expanded and its analysis is far more nuanced and balanced than were its early drafts. This change

is largely due, I believe, to the council's diligent efforts to solicit input
from a wide variety of stakeholders, including representatives of the
infertility advocacy and reproductive medicine communities, as well
as recognized legal and government experts. Since its formation, the
council has been the subject of extraordinary criticism about its com-
position and conduct. This report suggests that such concerns may
have been overblown. (Hudson 2004, 15)

Others argued similarly that the Kass Council produced both insightful
and balanced work (e.g., Rosen 2004; Smith 2003; McClay 2004).

Irrelevance

The council was tasked with providing fundamental inquiry in addition
to policy advice.[14] The substance and holism of its work, however, sparked
charges of irrelevance. Critics complained that the council's humanities-
based reflection was not pertinent to the practical demands of science
policy, where the scale of innovation, the pace of decisions, and the scope
of commercialization conspire to drown out fundamental inquiry (e.g.,
Nature Biotechnology 2003; Groopman 2002). One commentator called
the Kass Council "our first National Endowment for Rumination" (Ferguson 2002, 149).

Leigh Turner (2003) argued that the emphasis on philosophical reflection skewed the council's agenda toward an exclusive focus on novel biomedical science and technologies. This focus in turn removed attention
from pressing social issues related to bioethics, especially concerns about
public health and about the injustices created by the rising cost of healthcare. For example, Turner argued:

The council is looking at several rather speculative concerns instead
of addressing urgent matters . . . A body of this stature ought to focus
on issues of national and international importance. By limiting itself almost exclusively to advances in biomedical sciences and technology, and ignoring broader social issues, the council risks promoting a "bread and circuses" approach that entertains with the spectacle
of enhanced bodies and immortal lives but offers little meaningful
and substantive ethical analysis. (Turner 2003, 629)

Bioethicist Jonathan Moreno argued that the council should move "beyond the sexy biotech issues to those often collected under the rubric of justice" (Moreno 2005, 15; see also Lustig 2005). Journalist William Saletan (2004) implied that the council should be more like its member Fukuyama, who believes in "doing things" and "thinks the sex of intellectual exchange really is for the procreation of policy." Indeed, both Gazzaniga (2006) and Fukuyama (2005) argued that the Kass Council barely made a noticeable impact on federal legislation.[15]

Others defended the council's approach to bioethical inquiry (e.g., Asch 2005). Prior to her appointment to the council, Diana Schaub (in a review of the cloning report) celebrated the virtue of "contemplating one's navel," in the sense that the council meditated on the human core and deepened our self-understanding by reflecting on matters often overlooked (Schaub 2003, 50). Hudson argued that the real value of ethics advisory committees is often less in their recommendations, which are frequently ignored, than in "the manner and scope of their inquiry and the public discourse that they foster" (Hudson 2004, 15). A survey of bioethics committees around the world noted that their most important contributions are often their intangible efforts to "enhance the debate between science, the world of politics and the public" (Fuchs 2005, 92). Applying this general remark to the *Beyond Therapy* report, Elliott (2004) argued that the council had made a revolutionary contribution to public thought and policy discourse even though the report lacked any specific recommendations.

This issue came forward during the Kass Council's final meeting. There, Meilaender argued that the council was at its best when it did not focus on specific policy recommendations: "For me the most satisfying moments have been when we haven't worried about whether we're going actually to accomplish something in a policy sort of sense but have simply tried to sort through a question and say something about it." Meilaender likened the council's work to liberal education with the goals of reflective inquiry, critical thinking, and the formation of good character traits.

Council member Gómez-Lobo agreed with Meilaender by taking issue with the report by the Warnock Committee, a British bioethics commission on human fertilization and embryology chaired by analytic philosopher Mary Warnock. Fukuyama had earlier pointed to the Warnock report as a model for advisory bodies providing sound regulatory advice.

Gómez-Lobo, however, called the Warnock report "philosophically shallow" and in need of much greater reflection. It may have had a greater policy impact than the council's reports on the same topic, but Gómez-Lobo defended the greater philosophical depth of the Kass Council's work, which allowed for a deeper discussion and more cogent analysis. As Glendon put it during the final council session, "We have kept that tension alive, that theory and practice are, indeed, the two blades of the scissors and you cannot make a pleasing construction without using both of them" (September 9, 2005).

SIX

The Politicization of Ethics Advice

There is more at stake in the debate surrounding the "politicization" of the Kass Council than the fate of a single
advisory body. Indeed, this debate provides a perfect case
study to investigate the norms governing the interface between expert knowledge and democratic decision making.
The use of knowledge, especially scientific and technical
knowledge, to direct and justify action is intrinsic to liberal democratic notions of authority, accountability, and
order (Ezrahi 1990). But even as society comes to rely more
and more on experts to manage an increasingly technological society, it is far from clear precisely how the relationship between knowledge and power should be arranged (see
e.g., Bimber 1996). Throughout the modern era, proposals have ranged from complete autonomy for knowledge-
producers—usually scientists—to absolute control by political elites.

For reasons of freedom and accountability, neither of
these extremes is compatible with democracy. The production of knowledge must be both sheltered from and connected to society, and it is this delicate balance that the story
of the Kass Council can throw into relief. In examining this
issue, I hope to replace muddy terminology with clear standards. For example, Fletcher and Miller argue that the greatest peril of public bioethics is "political co-optation," which
"distorts ethical reflection" (Fletcher and Miller 1996, 157).

But "distorts" is too vague a term. It is better to see this politicization as the loss of democratic legitimacy stemming from actual and/or perceived failure to uphold the relevant norms of independence, balance, and transparency. The deligitimation of the Kass Council, which happened for several reasons, indicates how the idea of rich public bioethics could be better implemented in the future.

From Truth to Expertise: Legitimation of Special Knowledge in a Constructivist Age

In the "first wave" of science studies, when logical positivism reigned supreme, science was pictured as a value-free realm of truth (Collins and Evans 2006). We should trust or assent to the cognitive authority of scientists because they have special access to the truth. The current "second wave" of science studies has deflated this image of science.[1] The reality of scientific advisory bodies involves a murkier process than Truth speaking to Power (Jasanoff 1990). Oftentimes the experts do not agree amongst themselves. Decision making is forward-looking, so there is almost always uncertainty about the accuracy of scientific findings and predictions (Pielke 2007). Issues such as climate change and contraception involve values that will not be cleared away simply by "getting the science right" or "letting the science speak." Science can actually hamper policy making by creating an "excess of objectivity," or situations in which more than one theory can give an equally reasonable account of the relevant state of affairs (Sarewitz 2004).

The "second wave" of the systematic study of science has demystified scientific expertise. Thus, H. M. Collins and Robert Evans ask, "If it is no longer clear that scientists and technologists have special access to the truth, why should their advice be specially valued?" (Collins and Evans 2006, 40). When it comes to government advisory bodies or "public-domain sciences," rather than esoteric sciences, we cannot get by either with "first wave" blind trust or an equation of science with ideology. The first approach trades popular sovereignty for technocracy and has long proven an unacceptable response to the "principle-agent" dilemma posed by special knowledge in democratic societies (Guston 2000). The second approach devalues the important contributions of experts. Since government is involved with public-domain science, the relevant audience is broadened beyond the borders of any dispute among experts or over the credentialing process within a specialty to include at the very least some set of policy makers and perhaps even the public at large.

Legitimacy and Ethics Advice

Public advisory bodies are thus subject to processes of democratic legitimation. Democratic legitimacy often refers to popular acceptance of an authority. I use the term "legitimation" to refer to the processes and norms by which advisory bodies are granted popular assent or trust. By "legitimacy" I mean "a generalized perception or assumption that the actions of an entity are desirable, proper, or appropriate within some socially constructed system of norms, values, beliefs, and definitions" (Suchman 1995, 574). In other words, legitimacy is "the social acceptance resulting from adherence to regulative, normative or cognitive norms and expectations" (Deephouse and Carter 2005, 332). I take "delegitimation" to mean the loss of social acceptance resulting from perceived and/or actual failures to uphold the relevant norms.

Processes of democratic legitimation are crucial in structuring the giving of public advice, because effectively harnessing expertise for decision making requires managing public trust (Jasanoff 1990; Hilgartner 2000). Legitimacy is an intrinsic property and a social attribution. It is not possible to determine the legitimacy of an advisory body by isolating it from its social context and investigating how well it upholds the relevant norms, although this is part of the picture. Because legitimacy is about social acceptance, an advisory body's level of legitimacy will depend on perceptions. Thus an advisory body can—by all measures a researcher devises—excel in upholding the relevant norms but still lack legitimacy if opponents successfully tarnish its image with unfounded or vague accusations. It will be regarded suspiciously by relevant audiences, who will consequently refuse to engage its processes or treat its outcomes as credible—in short, it will be delegitimated.[2] When an organization is delegitimated, audiences suspect that "putatively efficacious procedures are tricks, or that putatively genuine structures are facades" (Suchman 1995, 597).

Some of the accusations challenging the legitimacy of the council can be proven wrong by showing them to be mischaracterizations. But even such false accusations, if they gain wide support, are instances of delegitimation. In addition to any faults on its part, there were contextual reasons why it was difficult for the council to maintain legitimacy. An advisory body working in a vitriolic political environment and within an administration itself suffering from credibility problems will be more vulnerable to attacks on its legitimacy than one working within more favorable circumstances. Furthermore, there is no way to guard against gratuitous attacks on an advisory body's legitimacy from ideologically motivated groups. Although they can do much to cultivate legitimacy, advisory bodies are ultimately not in control of their own fates.

Ethics and science advisory bodies are governed by the same procedures and norms, and they generate the same outcomes—deliberation and guidance on policy options.[3] Thus, democratic legitimation is at least as relevant for ethics advisory bodies as it is for science advisory bodies. Indeed, it is both more important and more difficult for ethics advisory bodies to secure legitimacy. This is due to popular perceptions that ethical inquiry is more "subjective" than scientific inquiry and thus more prone to political capture, raising the specter of "philosopher kings," arguably the antithesis of liberal democracy (see Dahl 1998).

Michael Walzer (1981) argues that ethics experts must practice "philosophic restraint." As with scientific advice, we often must settle not for the "right" answer, but for a better understanding, a clearer articulation of the stakes, and a more systematic subjection of alternatives to the trial of reasoned analysis, resulting in a "critically examined moral perspective" (Yoder 1998). Even if one thinks that there is no "right" answer to the kinds of issues the council investigated, one can still expect that, with the aid of experts, we can get a better understanding of different ways of assessing the relevant options and the merits for and against different courses of action.[4] The degree of help we can expect from the experts depends not only on their skills, but also on their legitimacy, which will determine whether the relevant audiences engage with their work.

The rise of modern science offered the promise that knowledge could rationalize politics. Yet the historical record justifies more pessimism than optimism on this score (see chapter 7). An instrumental-scientific conception of public action is insufficient. Bioethics committees, particularly those of the Kass Council's rich persuasion, can be seen as one instantiation of the resulting trend to deinstrumentalize public action by seeking knowledge about proper motivations, goals, and values, not only about efficient means. As I will argue further in the next chapter, such issues are intrinsic to public policy, despite the dream that social issues might become technical matters of utility maximization in which values disputes could be effectively bracketed.

Where scientific knowledge threatens to instrumentalize liberal democracy, ethical knowledge may threaten the traditional authority of science as public advisor. It may also be perceived as paternalistic—indeed the literature on bioethics committees demonstrates that a common concern is that ethics "experts" will dictate how people ought to live. The legitimacy of ethics advisory bodies is, then, doubly vulnerable: they will be open to general public skepticism about any admixture of liberal democracy with ethics experts, and rich versions in particular will be exposed to attacks from scientists challenging the value or validity of ethical knowledge. Together with the seemingly insurmountable partisanship of American politics, these realities will make the implemention of a rich public bioethics capable of fostering an inclusive conversation exceedingly difficult.

Norms of Legitimacy for the Kass Council and Politicization

Legitimacy is the social acceptance that results from being and being perceived as upholding certain norms and expectations, which serve as standards by which to judge the appropriate structure and behavior of advisory bodies. For judging the Kass Council, three norms are most important: independence, transparency, and balance.

These standards are codified in the 1972 Federal Advisory Committees Act (FACA), which requires oversight and accountability mechanisms for advisory bodies. It states that federal advisory committees are to be "fairly balanced in terms of the points of view represented and the functions to be performed by the advisory committee," and that their processes must "contain appropriate provisions to ensure that advice and recommendations . . . will not be inappropriately influenced by the appointing authority or by any special interest, but will instead be the result of the advisory committee's independent judgment" (FACA, 5 U.S.C. Appendix 2, Section 5(b) 2 and 3). There is also a statute on conflicts of interest (18 U.S.C. § 208) that is enforced by the Office of Government Ethics (OGE). Furthermore, advisory committee meetings and transcripts are mandated to be open to the public.

That these are the relevant norms is further indicated by a report issued by the General Accounting Office (USGAO 2004). Furthermore, Kass promised that the council should act according to these norms (see Cameron 2002, 44). And at the first council meeting, he remarked that the council should "consult very widely and . . . hear from the various people with different interests and different points of view . . . These positions [are to] show the effects of having engaged the other side of the conversation so that one is not simply talking with preconceived notions but that our deliberations would, in fact, issue in the best possible statements of whatever points of view are germane to the issue" (January 17, 2002).

Council reports provide further evidence that it was claiming to uphold these norms. For example, in its cloning report the council argued for the importance of a representative and fair discussion of the issues (Kass Council 2003a, 121–22). All these points suggest that balance, independence, and transparency are appropriate expectations for the council and appropriate norms by which to judge its level of democratic legitimacy.[5]

We are now in a position to examine claims about "politicization," which is a term widely used and rarely defined. I take politicization to mean a certain type of delegitimation, one in which the norms defended above are or are perceived to be eroded by inappropriate partisanship. This definition distinguishes politicization from other ways in which legitimacy can be undermined (e.g., actual or perceived incompetence). The council was politicized in the sense that it was widely perceived as failing to uphold the pertinent norms due to partisanship. Council opponents were successful in diverting a substantive discussion about bioethics issues into a political battle about the legitimacy of the council. This leaves open the question of whether and at what points the council was in fact acting in the ways that many perceived or accused it to be. In other words, to what extent and when were charges of politicization and/or defenses against such charges ploys in political strategies rather than fair appraisals of the council?

My use of the term "politicization" lacks the positive connotations of its use where "politics" is understood as "the activity of ordering our lives together" (Cohen 2004). In that sense, the politicization of science, technology, and ethics is an essential good for democratic societies as public reasoning is openly brought to bear on matters that impact all citizens. The negative sense of politicization works to undermine the positive sense by discrediting potential sources of useful knowledge and potential forums of civil, informed debate. My use of the term is also more specific than the more general usage, according to which bioethics is politicized as soon as it becomes entangled with power relations, and mechanisms must be found for facilitating dialogue, negotiating interests, and resolving disagreements (see Brown 2008). Indeed, my usage helps distinguish between better and worse ways to "politicize" bioethics in this broader sense.

Perceived Politicization: The Kass Council as Stealth Advocate?

In his analysis of science policy, Roger Pielke (2007) imagines he is new to town and in need of advice on where to eat lunch. He turns for advice to the attendant at the local information kiosk; as a resident and a tourist bureau official, she seems like a trustworthy source of information. He tells her the kind of food he likes and sets a price range. She in turn lays out several options. This is how we expect an expert to perform in such situations—multiplying a range of relevant options and providing reason-giving accounts of their pros and cons in light of our goals. Pielke calls this type of expert the "honest broker of policy alternatives." The same aim could be accomplished in another way by assembling the managers of many restaurants and having them each present a sales pitch. Here the expert is working to reduce options to one preferred outcome. Pielke calls this kind of expert the "issue advocate."

An ethics advisory body could follow either model and still be capable of securing democratic legitimacy. We could imagine a panel of ethicists each espousing different arguments about a biomedical research project, or we could imagine a panel of ethics experts who each play the role of analyst weighing all options. Actual ethics advisory bodies mix both models. Importantly, however, when the advocacy model is employed, the chair or the committee as a whole must work as a synthesizing analyst to give each position a fair hearing when publishing reports.

Introducing a third model of expertise will help explain how the Kass Council was politicized in the eyes of many. Imagine now that the information kiosk attendant is only masquerading as a tourist bureau official when she is in fact a sales representative for one particular restaurant. There are many ways she could bias your decision in favor of her restaurant. She could leave other options out, mischaracterize them, downplay other restaurants and hype hers, etc. She is pretending to be an honest broker when in fact she is playing the role of an advocate. I call this role the expert as "stealth advocate."[6] A special or partisan interest takes the guise of an analyst focused on the common interest (the advice seeker here symbolizing an elected policy maker seeking the common good). Or, we could imagine a supposedly balanced and diverse panel of advocates that is in reality a homogenous group favoring the same foregone conclusion. This wolf-in-sheep's-clothing scenario is the best way to understand the accusations that the Kass Council was politicized.

Critics maintained that the council only masqueraded as an honest broker, when it should have at the very least admitted to being an advocate. I listed numerous examples of this kind of criticism in the last chapter. There we also saw that others defended the council's legitimacy. (None of the defenders advanced the argument that ethics advisory bodies do not need democratic legitimacy. Rather, all claimed that the critics were mistaken in their portrayals of the council.)

The outcome of these disputes was a general erosion of the council's legitimacy, as its tenure was dominated by political controversy rather than substantive debates about its work. Many successful critics adopted the rhetoric of disinterested science to effectively undermine the council from an authoritative and supposedly "neutral" position. Yet as the following evaluation will show, some criticisms of the council were accurate. Thus, the council was in part responsible for its own flagging legitimacy. All of this highlights a need for improving future ethics advisory committees, especially their rules and procedures for mission creation, membership appointment, report publication, and member behavior.

Actual Politicization? Three Case Studies from the Kass Council

In what follows, I attempt a reasonable assessment of the council, judging events in light of the guiding norms. Applying these standards requires context-sensitive analysis by triangulating and weighing sources of information to the greatest extent possible. Many accusations centered on three events involving the council and its members. A focus on these may bias an evaluation in the direction of a less favorable assessment, but it also directs attention to the most salient potential problems.

Blackburn Purged for Not Conforming?

On February 27, 2004, the White House notified council member Elizabeth Blackburn that she had not been reappointed to the council at the end of her first two-year term, which came as a surprise to her (Blackburn 2004a; 2004b). Though she had worked on the report *Reproduction and Responsibility* and prepared a personal statement, her remarks were not published and her name was not listed among the authors. Upon her release, accusations flew, including one remark that "Kass has his commission under control" after purging a "pro–stem cell" member (Kennedy 2004).

Blackburn claimed that she was dismissed because she disagreed with Kass and President Bush on the ethics of stem cell research and cloning. She maintained that they had narrowed the diversity of views crucial to good bioethics advice. Many (e.g., Michaels et al. 2002; UCS 2004; Waxman 2004) argued this was part of a pattern of the Bush administration seeking "advice without dissent." Some 170 researchers signed an open letter to Bush protesting the decision and the American Society for Cell Biology, representing 11,000 scientists, issued a public statement denouncing Blackburn's dismissal as an affront to the norms of federal advice-seeking (ASCB 2004; Holden 2004).

Kass claimed the release of Blackburn signified only a shift in focus from reproduction and genetics to issues of neuroscience, brain, and behavior. He remarked, "Unfortunately, these membership changes were met with unfounded and false charges of political 'stacking' of the council . . . We shall continue to honor the diversities of our views, confident that the reports we write will contribute to public understanding and earn the re-spect of fair-minded readers" (Kass 2004).

Legitimacy is lost if members are selected in order to represent only one political view or dismissed because their views differ from those of the president or the chair. (In some cases members can be selected according to political views if this process culminates in a diversity of such views.) Just as importantly, a legitimate panel cannot be formed if there is wide-spread suspicion of such practices. In order for Blackburn and other crit-ics to support their argument they first needed to show that her replace-ment held views sympathetic to those of Bush. Blackburn did claim that the three replacements[7] were a neurosurgeon who championed religious values in public life (Carson), a political scientist who publicly praised Kass (Schaub), and a political philosopher who described as "evil" any research that destroys embryos (Lawler) (Union of Concerned Scientiests 2004).

Benjamin Carson was the neurosurgeon who officially replaced Black-burn. Blackburn noted his openly Christian life-philosophy, which was ap-parent in his speeches and books (e.g., Carson 1992). Kass (2004) referred to him as a "keen booster of science and medical advance," which is ap-parent based on his neurosurgery publications, honorary degrees, and na-tional citations of merit. Even if we admit that Carson and the other re-placements were sympathetic to Bush's views, the more difficult element in proving misconduct is to establish that they were hired for this rea-son. Otherwise it is just as reasonable to accept Kass's explanation for the change, because subsequent council meetings did address neuroscience, which is Carson's expertise. Here the accusations drift into speculation. On one hand, Kass's remarks about the new members' personal views being "completely unknown" to him is doubtful. But on the other hand, why was Blackburn dismissed instead of Gazzaniga or Janet Rowley, who were ar-guably more vocally antithetical to Kass's views? Rowley coauthored a pub-lication with Blackburn accusing Kass of stacking the council, but she was not released.

But this is not to dismiss the critics' charges. In fact, the reason for speculation is the closed nature of the (re)appointment process. Even if the charges are off the mark (i.e., they do not accurately reflect Kass's and Bush's intentions), the secretive nature of the process contributes to skep-ticism and eventual weakening of legitimacy. So the perceived lack of independence and balance is partially caused and aggravated by an actual lack of transparency.

While this lack of transparency may not violate the letter of the law, it violates the spirit of the law that mandates openness for council meetings and certain electronic transactions. In fact, a suspicion that there was something indecent transpiring on the "backstage" (cf. Hilgartner 2000) of the council delegitimated it in the eyes of some from before the first meeting, because the original selection of members, including Kass, was highly secretive (Caplan 2002; Gillespie 2002). The suspicion of an off-the-record process played a role in controversies around its cloning report (see Hall 2002[8]). Accusations arose that a small coalition, led by Kass, altered the report behind closed doors without consent by all members.[9]

Accusations of political influence and lack of balance in membership are not unprecedented. Al Jonsen (1998) noted that the appointment of new members to a previous bioethics committee (the President's Commission) led to substantial changes in its report *Securing Access to Health Care*. In the early 1980s, ten members who had been appointed by President Carter were replaced with members agreeable to conservative Republican views. Thus Blackburn was certainly not the first to leave a bioethics commission, but she may have been the first to be replaced by the same administration after a single term of service because of her views. Although, again, it is not clear if this was the reason for her dismissal.

The Misuse of Science or No Chance for Dissent?

Blackburn maintained that her dismissal was precipitated by the article she coauthored with Rowley (Blackburn and Rowley 2004). She claimed she was dismissed after showing it to Kass. In it, Blackburn and Rowley critique two of the council's reports, *Beyond Therapy* and *Monitoring Stem Cell Research*. Their complaint has two components: the first claim is that Kass and the council misused science, while the second claim is that Kass made a promise about the fair inclusion of dissenting voices in council reports that he failed to uphold.

Defining criteria for the misuse of science is difficult in the abstract. Pielke (2004), however, identifies a type of misuse, "mischaracterization," that reflects Blackburn and Rowley's accusations. Mischaracterization is the incorrect or misleading representation of a research report or particular finding. It can include overhyping the promises of or the perils from pursuing or avoiding a particular line of research. Judging when mischaracterization has occurred requires significant interpretation and clarity about what counts as a proper characterization of the science.

Blackburn and Rowley do not provide this level of analysis in their accusations. Many of their complaints are about the interpretation of facts (or uncertainties) and the conclusions drawn from them; the selection of some information and omission of other information; and the tone of the reports. But in none of these cases do they differentiate between the unethical misuse of science and the inevitable need of the council to make decisions and compromises about exclusions, omissions, and emphases in group-authored reports.

For example, Blackburn and Rowley complained about the specter of designer babies raised in *Beyond Therapy.* They argued that the report does not adequately clarify the unlikelihood of this possibility: "While such scientific unlikelihood is mentioned in passing in the report, it is easy to take away from the report the feeling that such genetic manipulation will happen and is even imminent" (Blackburn and Rowley 2004, 420). Yet *Beyond Therapy* states, "But in our considered judgment, these dreams of fully designed babies, based on directed genetic change, are for the foreseeable future pure fantasies . . . Straightforward genetic engineering of better children may prove impossible, not only in practice but even in principle" (Kass Council 2003a, 37–38). These lines throw into doubt the accusation that the report gives the kind of impression that Blackburn and Rowley claimed.

Blackburn and Rowley noted that the inclusion of a "sensational quote" by one researcher in *Beyond Therapy* leads to a "misleading misrepresentation of the motivation of reputable researchers in the field of aging" (Blackburn and Rowley 2004, 420). But this quote is in a footnote that acknowledges this very concern (Kass Council 2003a, 162). Their complaints about the stem cell report were "that some facts that would help the public and scientists better assess the content of the report were not brought out clearly or were omitted entirely" (Blackburn and Rowley 2004, 421). But the first evidence they cite involves not "facts" but the distillation of a "major message" from the peer-reviewed literature, namely, that there is a vast difference between our understanding of adult and of embryonic stem cells. They state that it is important to emphasize a point about multi-potent adult progenitor cells (MAPCs) that is included verbatim in the report (Kass Council 2004a, 124), but deserves additional commentary according to Blackburn and Rowley (Blackburn and Rowley 2004, 421). They conclude that the science was distorted and presented incompletely, but they do not differentiate the necessary tasks of editing and interpreting from the unethical act of mischaracterizing.

Blackburn and Rowley did not provide solid evidence that science was misused. Their complaints were primarily about where emphasis should be placed, what voices should be included in the report, and what interpretations should be given to the scientific literature. But though they are unable to prove in broad terms that science had been misused, the second element of their complaint is more easily substantiated and more amenable to targeted reforms of future committees.

Blackburn and Rowley do explicitly formulate the second complaint, writing that "we were persuaded [by Kass] that our voices would be heard and integrated into statements of the Council," but that Kass failed to live up to this promise (2004, 420). This accusation amounts to the charge that within the bounds of reasonable interpretations of the science (i.e., not mischaracterizations) all opinions, including minority dissensions, should be included in final reports that present the public voice of the council. This complaint is not about properly characterizing the science; rather it pertains to the rules for including reasonable differences about how to interpret, emphasize, edit, and contextualize vast bodies of knowledge in the creation of an advisory report.

In order to substantiate this claim, it must first be shown that Kass did promise council members that the council would respect and represent diverse opinions. Although we cannot verify private conversations between Kass, Blackburn, and Rowley, there are two other sources that support the claim that Blackburn and Rowley were justified in expecting all voices to be represented in formal reports. First, the executive order reads: "The Council shall be guided by the need to articulate fully the complex and often competing moral positions on any given issue, rather than by an overriding concern to find consensus. The council may therefore choose to proceed by offering a variety of views on a particular issue, rather than attempt to reach a single consensus position." Second, in his open-ing remarks, Kass stated, "Because reasonable and morally serious people can differ about fundamental matters, it is fortunate that we have been lib-erated from an overriding concern to reach consensus . . . All serious rele-vant opinions, carefully considered, are welcome" (January 17, 2002).

Finally, to substantiate this claim it must be shown that Blackburn's and Rowley's voices were not adequately represented in these two reports. As mentioned earlier, the *Beyond Therapy* report does include some foot-notes that explicitly address council member disagreement (e.g., Kass Council 2003a, 162). But in the particular instance of the motivation of age-retardation research, for example, Blackburn and Rowley's concerns could have been mitigated by the inclusion of another quote from a differ-ent researcher in the field.

For the most part, there are not large differences between the state-ments Blackburn and Rowley would have liked to see in the stem cell re-port and the statements actually made in the report. But in its discussion of the state of stem cell research the report does not explicitly refer to differences of interpretation among council members. There is no vehicle for presenting dissent through footnotes, in-text commentary, or sepa-rate "minority report" sections. Indeed, unlike most of the council's other reports, both *Beyond Therapy* and *Monitoring Stem Cell Research* are no-ticeably deficient when it comes to conveying dissent. A more explicit in-clusion of such mechanisms would have helped mitigate conflict and per-ceptions of bias. For example, the stem cell report states, "Despite the fact that the [various adult] stem cell preparations used are not well character-ized, and reproducible results have yet to be obtained, preliminary find-ings are sometimes encouraging" (Kass Council 2004a, 126). This would have been a good comment to footnote with Blackburn and Rowley's in-terpretation that "many of the reports on the properties of cells differen-tiated from adult stem cell preparations are to date preliminary and in-complete" (Blackburn and Rowley 2004, 421).

These instances raise considerations of how advisory reports should be crafted in order to maintain transparency and the diverse balance of views necessary for legitimacy while still making the compromises that are of practical necessity in compiling and condensing information. For example, how should judgments be made about which scientific evidence to include and how it should be interpreted? Who should be in charge of determining whether the final report gives the right impression about the nature of potential problems or the state of the science? How should dissenting voices be represented and to what extent? How should advisory panels turn backstage debates into a coherent public document that all can own? These sorts of political and procedural questions are more fruitful to pursue than accusations of "distortion" that in this case devolved into a "scientization" of moral and political issues (Cook 2004).

A Conflict of Interest?

The first two controversies raised questions about appointment and reporting mechanisms. The final case examines standards of conduct for advisory panel members, especially their chairs. It was here that accusations of improper actions gained their greatest traction.

In 2005 a coalition of conservatives led by Kass released a document entitled "Bioethics for the Second Term: Legislative Recommendations." It proposed an "offensive bioethics agenda" comprised of recommendations to prohibit the "most egregious biotechnical advances" (Cohen 2005a). The document was controversial and even came under attack by conservatives such as Senator Sam Brownback (Weiss 2005). It was published as an editorial in the conservative-leaning journal *The New Atlantis*, some of whose editors (e.g., Eric Cohen and Yuval Levin) were council staffers.

Kass stressed that his involvement in this coalition was independent of his role as council chair and that no federal resources were used by the nameless conservative group. But some argued that Kass was trading on his position as chair to advance a narrow political agenda, constituting a conflict of interest (Pielke 2005; Murray 2005). I define "conflict of interest" in a political sense to mean when someone in a position of trust based in part on political independence takes on a partisan role that undermines confidence in his ability to fill his role as an independent broker. The accusation was that Kass adopted a position of advocacy that compromised his ability to maintain the role of analyst, crucial for the chair of an advisory body. The argument continued that Kass delegitimated the council by weakening his reputation as a broker of critical reflection and balanced analysis.

Iain Murray (2005) argued that legitimacy does not require all members of an advisory panel to be free from conflicts of interest. But it does require that the chair be as neutral as possible. The chair has the authority to shape debates and publications, and management for legitimacy requires that full and fair hearings be given to all reasonable competing sides. Legitimacy is possible in theory even if a chair holds his or her own views and argues for those views consistently while on a committee. But Kass was such an active chair (he devoted a great deal of his time to council duties, branding its work with his distinctive style) and controversial figure that the council's image was closely tied with his own. He could retain his own substantive views in council deliberations to some extent (providing that the synthetic work of an analyst is accomplished somehow), but to publicly adopt a partisan position would quite predictably identify the council with conservative politics in the minds of many people.

Council member James Wilson (2005) wrote a rebuttal to Murray's account, arguing that Kass's actions did not represent a conflict of interest and that his position as chair of the council would not make it more likely that his views would get more of a hearing than other well-qualified bioethicists. Yet Kass's "bioethics agenda" received press in both the *Washington Post* (Weiss 2005) and *Science* magazine (Kintisch 2005), which suggests that his position did leverage greater publicity. Wilson did not defend his assertion that there was no conflict of interest in Kass's actions with any arguments. A strong case thus remains that Kass's actions created a clear conflict of interest that further eroded the legitimacy of the council.

In summary, this brief evaluation suggests that there were some instances of actual politicization to justify some accusations. In other instances, however, the criticisms were off the mark and reflected more the polarized climate of American bioethics and politics than the actual structures and procedures of the council or behaviors of its members.

Who's to Blame?

The politicization of ethics advice in this case hurt the common interest by discrediting an otherwise capable forum for reflection on matters of public concern. An exhaustive assessment of politicization of the Kass Council would need to detail similar controversies surrounding the formation of the council, including its mission statement and membership selection as well as accusations that *Reproduction and Responsibility* reached consensus because dissent had been squelched through inappropriate backstage acts. But a closer look at these other issues will reveal the same need to secure independence, balance, and especially transparency. In these cases, legitimacy could have been enhanced through improved transparency of mission formation, membership selection, and report finalization.

Though my evaluation shows that he greatly overstates his claim, Leigh Turner does summarize well the importance of legitimacy and the consequences of its erosion:

> Credible advisory bodies benefit from broad bipartisan support; they gain legitimacy insofar as citizens from different cultural, political, religious and philosophical backgrounds view them as trustworthy and insightful. Thus, although conservatives on the Council might find deliberations easier with a panel loaded with clones of Kass, overall, their credibility is likely to be harmed by the perception that shared understandings have been achieved by excluding from the debate voices that belong in their deliberations. As a result, the capacity of the Council to speak in a common voice will only emerge at a moment when many concerned citizens have already ceased listening. (Turner 2004, 510)

As noted above, the political context made "broad bipartisan support" all but impossible. The council could hardly be blamed for failing to achieve it. Furthermore, as meeting transcripts (particularly those leading up to the cloning and stem cell reports) and published dissent in council reports demonstrate, the Kass Council was far from philosophically homogenous. But Turner is right to note that the council could have done more to bolster its own legitimacy by paying greater attention to the way it went about implementing the important ideal of a rich public bioethics.

The ability of the Kass Council to implement a rich public bioethics and achieve the goals of improved advice, discussion, and understanding hinged on the organizational details of the federal advisory process. This process and the institutions that embody it must skillfully shelter ethical or scientific inquiry from narrow partisanship while robustly connecting it to policy and the wider public sphere.

On one hand, as this analysis shows, the Kass Council bears some blame for its low level of legitimacy. In some cases, such as "stacking" its staff with contributors to conservative publications and even permitting staff members to openly defend "conservative bioethics," its practices appear to be intentional. Other cases seem to be the result of insufficient attention to structures and procedures. While in many cases the Kass Council exercised appropriate diligence in these matters—for example, in its careful deliberations to ensure inclusiveness and openness in its stem cell report (transcripts from October 17, 2003)—at other points, the council could have performed better. If one wants to engage society in bioethics inquiry, one cannot simply wish away politics. Attention must be paid to the details of managing legitimacy.

On the other hand, many council critics offered unsubstantiated and vague accusations, instead of reasoned analyses supported by empirical claims. In seeking to delegitimate the council by reducing it to partisan politics by other means, they diminished substantial engagements with the ideas put forth in council reports. This damage was the more severe, because it is precisely such thoughtful engagement that the public and decision makers most need in the face of complex bioethical quandaries. Many critics showed no concern for common interests and did not want the Kass Council to succeed on any metric. In such a context, not even a perfectly crafted advisory body would be able to achieve its goals. Ultimately, bioethics consultation, particularly novel forms of it such as the one adopted by the Kass Council, depends on open minds willing to engage in conversation.

SEVEN

The Kass Council as Humanities Policy

Nathaniel Hawthorne's short story "The Birth-mark" tells of a scientist, Aylmer, who becomes obsessed with his beautiful wife's only blemish. His growing disgust at the small hand-shaped birthmark on her cheek shames his wife, Georgiana, and persuades her to cooperate with his plan to remove it. Yet in trying to erase the stigma, and despite all the secrets of his "deep science," Aylmer causes Georgiana's death. The story is profoundly ethical in portraying a man who is unhappy because the world does not meet the conditions he lays down. We see in concrete detail the destruction of life, beauty, and goodness that results from Aylmer's attitude toward the world.

At its first meeting, the Kass Council entered a discussion of this story in a session entitled "Science and the Pursuit of Perfection." Some members were silent during the discussion, indicating a protest both against the substance of the story and the unusual practice of literary hermeneutics as part of policy advice. Others outside of the council pounced on this episode as emblematic of the council's overall impracticality. The physician Jerome Groopman (2002), for example, could find no practical value in beginning "not with facts but with fiction." Indeed, as we saw in chapter 5, a major criticism of the Kass Council was that its rich humanistic inquiry was irrelevant to public policy.

In another example, the editors of *Nature Biotechnology* (2003), with palpable annoyance and exasperation, concluded their parody of *Beyond
Therapy*, entitled "Beyond Belief," with the chastisement: "There are times
for getting to the damn point."

In this chapter, I will use such charges of irrelevance to look beyond
bioethics and reflect on a central question of knowledge politics: what is
pertinent knowledge for public policy? Since World War II, policymakers
have increasingly viewed scientific and technical knowledge as central to
achieving societal goals. Groopman's comment indicates the basic idea: get
the facts—the science—right and problems will be solved. By contrast,
the humanities account for less than one percent of the public resources
invested in knowledge.[1] It is commonly held that the humanities have
at best a marginal role in addressing social challenges from health care to
defense to energy and environment. Bioethics commissions and similar
initiatives—for example, the ethical, legal, and social impacts (ELSI) research element of the human genome project and the national nanotech-
nology initiative—are the most notable exceptions.

Such utilizations of ethics and other humanities for public policy are
the result of a basic insight: many of the questions faced by high-tech societies are not themselves technological or scientific, but rather humanistic.
Part I provided numerous examples of such questions confronted by the
Kass Council, from the funding of embryonic stem cell research to the use
of pharmacological enhancements. The most pertinent knowledge, then,
is often that which pertains to the most ancient questions: How should we
live? What is a good and just society? Science can provide instrumental
knowledge about how to achieve different courses of action. But the humanities offer improved insight into the relative value of competing alternatives, thereby helping to identify desirable policy actions. I will call
such uses of the humanities for policy making "humanities policy."

If we are to see the novel contribution of the Kass Council, we will
need to maintain the distinction made in part I and differentiate between
an instrumentalist and a rich humanities policy. Indeed, the remark about
getting to the point encompasses an instrumentalist principle that expands
beyond bioethics. This instrumentalism conceives of policy making as a
machine for processing inputs (knowledge and interests) and outputs (decisions). Public policy making is a means-ends operation. It has a "point,"

and the object is to "get there." Apparent in this instrumentalism are its telltale isolationism and formalism. Policy making is a discrete sequence of problems isolated from culture, history, psychology, and philosophy. The interests that clash around these problems are fixed and uneducable.

Instrumentalist humanities policy does not question this image of policy. Rather, the humanities are utilized as inputs — in addition to science — to fill existing policy vacuums and resolve ethical dilemmas. On this view, ethics advisory bodies act as instruments for enhancing the performance of the machine. This metaphor is presumed by studies that measure the "impact" of advisory bodies (see Wolanin 1975; Ellen, Bobby, and Fineberg 1995; Eiseman 2003). In its formulation of principles for research with human subjects, the Belmont Report issued by the National Commission scores high on such impact analyses. As we saw in chapter 3, the Kass Council also produced policy principles and recommendations capable of being plugged into the policy process. This is an important function of advisory bodies. Thus, like instrumental bioethics, policy instrumentalism is one viable and important conceptual framework.

But it is also incomplete in ways that distort a full understanding of what policy making and politics are and thus the wider possible contributions of the humanities. According to instrumentalism, if there is no immediate discernable "impact," then the advisory work was a failure. But this cannot be the only metric of relevance, especially considering how little control advisory bodies have over the political fate of their work.[2] Indeed, another, deeper, contribution of the humanities becomes apparent only by questioning the instrumentalist notion of policy. Rich humanist inquiry helps us to see policy as more than an isolated machine for matching means and ends within a clash of fixed interests. True to its holism and substance, rich inquiry casts policy making within wider contexts in which "interests" are formed and re-formed, in part by critically reflecting on and expanding human values and sympathies. Much that is central to policy consists in the longer historical timeline and the broader cultural context of contesting and figuring out what the "point" is, not simply getting there.

In what follows, I will first demonstrate the insufficiency of a purely scientific and technical public policy instrumentalism. My focus is on "science policy" contexts broadly understood as the production and utilization of science in government decisions (science for policy) and decisions directing the production of science (policy for science). I will then briefly discuss the merits of incorporating the humanities into an otherwise unchanged policy instrumentalism. My emphasis, however, will be to draw inspiration from the Kass Council's use of literature—especially in its report *Being Human*—in order to demonstrate the relevance of a rich humanities policy.

The Rise and Fall of Instrumentalism in Science for Policy

For Machiavelli, Hobbes, and other early moderns, politics was conceptualized as a human enterprise exposed to the disruption of *fortuna,* or contingent forces. The political order was understood as a human construction designed to secure pleasure and minimize pain. The principle constraint on realizing such goals was not a supernatural will, but rather nature, or, more proximally, our limited capacity for understanding, predicting, and controlling nature, including the nature of individual humans and societies. Applied scientific knowledge, therefore, has since grown into the crucial guide for political action. With this ascendance of science, the once privileged role of moral knowledge and virtue in the political order declined. Politics became less a matter of perfecting citizens than of skillfully using knowledge as an instrument to achieve given, desired ends. As Machiavelli argued in the dedication to the foundational work of modern republicanism, esteem should be granted to those who know how to govern states, rather than to those who have the right to govern, but lack the knowledge (*Discourses* 1513).

This instrumental conception of politics bolstered arguments, such as those put forward by Henri de Saint-Simon, for technocracy, wherein an elite class of experts can manage society through their specialized technical knowledge. But as Yaron Ezrahi notes, a more important trend was the combination of the instrumental notion of politics with a commitment to freedom and democracy. Since the rise of modern natural science, "the role of knowledge and technique in directing and justifying action has become central to modern Western liberal-democratic notions of authority, accountability, and order" (Ezrahi 1990, 3). Liberal democracies do not use science only to enhance their effectiveness in achieving goals—they rely on scientific knowledge to legitimate their modes of political action and claims to power.

The nineteenth century witnessed the rise of utopian visions of science rationalizing democracy, carrying politics on its wings above scarcity, conflict, and chance. Scientific discourses from physics to physiology were extended from nature to society (see Olson 2008). They would replace myths, ideology, or authority with knowledge as the basis of social action. The zenith of the replacement of politics with technical rationality came in the early twentieth century. The "scientific management" of Frederick Winslow Taylor spread to matters of policy, for example, in the notion that forestry science could provide the "one best way" to manage public forests. Policy making is understood here as simply the identification and application of the most effective means to achieve given ends. Thus, the word "policy" came to connote an instrumentalist process of isolating problems and applying expert tools to solve them. The geneticist J. B. S. Haldane (1924) argued that the application of science to human problems would conquer not only nature, but even the "dark and evil elements" in the human soul.

Haldane was assuming an enlightenment metaphor of science as the mirror of nature (see Rorty 1979). The mirror metaphor justified the notion that science could cement diverse experiences into a single public reality, which would constrain the validity of claims made by actors in the social sphere. Yet over the course of the twentieth century, developments in science itself contributed to undermine this metaphor. The rise of Big Science with its complex instrumentation widened the rift between scientific and commonsense knowledge and between lay and professional concepts of evidence and proof. The increasing commercialization of science and instances of fraud further undermined the cultural authority of science (Greenberg 2001).

Most damaging to the mirror metaphor, however, was a growing realization that interpretation, uncertainty, and disagreement are intrinsic to science. Quantum physicists were among the first to articulate a new metaphor of science. For example, Werner Heisenberg (1952), drawing from Goethe, noted that the experiments of physicists do not disclose "nature itself," but rather a nature that is transformed through the course of research. He further argued that science is not built on a "rock-like foundation" but is rather "suspended over an unfathomable depth." Nature as we know it, even through science, is not independent of cognition, but is a product of the interaction between humans and the world. Seeing is a form of constructing and interpreting, not simply mirroring. John Dewey calls this a shift from the "spectator" theory of knowledge to one of active participation. This shift took a relativist turn in constructivist camps that sought to knock science off of its privileged epistemological vantage point.

The instrumental rationalization of politics, which had reached prominence in "cost-benefit analyses" and other "policy analyses," began to draw fire in the wake of this shift. James March and Herbert Simon pointed out that "classical" economic and organizational theories failed to recognize the subjective character of rationality and the fact that politics is far more a game of "satisficing" than "maximizing" goods. Kenneth Arrow (1951) argued that there are no value-neutral or instrumental rules for deriving public welfare from diverse individual preferences. There is an irreducible nonscientific, value-laden core to any "collective rationality." Charles Lindblom (1959) and Aaron Wildavsky (1964) similarly critiqued the "rational-comprehensive" approach to public policy as a supposedly value-free, instrumental matching of means and ends.

Later analyses showed how the instrumentalization of politics can actually exacerbate rather than solve problems (e.g., Sarewitz 2004). As Roger Pielke (2007) notes, "getting the science right" compels action only in contexts where uncertainty and values disputes are minimal. Where there is uncertainty and disagreement—which is true of most public policy issues—science can actually further muddle the situation. The reason for this is twofold. First, the failure of science to mirror nature produces an "excess of objectivity" (Sarewitz 1997). In complex systems, it is not possible to get a unified view of the world as it really is. Different scientists—in good faith—paint different pictures. Second, the iron triangle of politicians, scientists, and special interest groups produce a multiplicity of scientifically based policies. Politicians try to avoid hard decisions that could upset parts of their constituencies. Instead they fund scientists to "figure it out," and the scientists are happy to oblige. This research inevitably creates an "excess of objectivity," which means that special interest advocates can cherry-pick the experts who support their views. The upshot is that explicit policy debate about values is replaced with political gridlock in the guise of (supposedly value-free) science.[3] The same dynamic is visible in supposedly value-free bioethics.

Criticisms of the mirror metaphor and instrumentalism have given rise to "postnormal" science and politics (e.g., Funtowicz and Ravetz 1993). This approach sees politics as increasingly fragmented, heterogeneous, symbolic, and incoherent. At the same time, science becomes less a universal legitimizing discourse than ammunition in commercial ventures and political disputes. Citizens become less passive witnesses to the actions of scientists (mediated through "fact" or "reality") than active participants co-constructing claims within political-scientific dramas. Science becomes "democratized" through greater access, awareness, and participation (e.g., Dickson 1984; Sclove 1995).

One response to postnormal science policy is a pervasive skepticism: politics is seen simply as the bargaining of fixed, preestablished interests, and science is seen as politics by other means. Here the boundaries of rationality collapse as both epistemic and ethical norms are taken to be culturally relative.[4] Humanities policy initiatives such as bioethics commissions, however, represent another possible response. They expand the boundaries of rationality to include ethics and other aspects of the human sciences, rather than collapsing them. Indeed, the most pertinent knowledge for public action often entails inquiry into values, goals, and motivations, not just efficient means.

The Rise and Fall of Instrumentalism in Policy for Science

The instrumentalism above took the form of a utopian myth that value-laden politics could be replaced by expert scientific rationality. The instrumentalism discussed in this section is a predominant trend in a science policy that seeks the best means to the assumed ends of economic growth and technological innovation. Again, these ends—such as safety, justice, and autonomy in instrumental bioethics—are not the wrong ones to pursue. They are, however, limited; that is, high-tech societies with large GDPs are not necessarily just societies and do not necessarily foster happiness, well-being, and virtue in their citizens. A problem occurs when

an emphasis on economy and technology is overextended to the exclu-
sion of broader considerations.

World War II was a watershed for U.S. science policy.[5] Prior to the war,
physicists were nearly as unemployable as philosophers are today. In 1932
the U.S. federal government devoted 0.35 percent of its national income to
research and development. By 1962 that figure had grown an order of mag-
nitude to three percent, a much bigger slice of a bigger pie (Brooks 1996).
In another sign of this remarkable development, by 1965 U.S. ambassador to the United Nations Adlai Stevenson could suggest that science and
technology were more important to policy than anything else because
they "are making the problems of today irrelevant in the long run."

In his 1945 report to the U.S. president, *Science—The Endless Frontier,* Vannevar Bush sought to justify wartime levels of funding for science during times of peace. Bush formulated what has come to be known
as the "linear model" of science-society relations. It articulates two theses: (a) basic research leads to applied research and technologies in a linear fashion; and (b) this process occurs best when scientists are granted
autonomy from political forces. This position involves a central paradox:
research performed without any thought of practical benefits is justified
by its practical benefits—and excused from responsibility for any bad
outcomes that result (Pielke and Byerly 1998). The conception of basic
research leading automatically and directly to the betterment of society
took hold, not in strong institutional forms, but in the minds of many of
those involved in science policy (Stokes 1997).

This means in practice that science policy is primarily science *budget*
policy. The focus of those who make and analyze science policies is largely
on questions of monetary *inputs* into research and development. Yet much
of science policy research and practice[6] has since become an extended and
increasingly critical analysis of the linear model and its oftentimes inadequate views. These analyses all share an emphasis on *outputs,* which in turn
requires a greater understanding of the processes by which investments in
research translate into societal results. Thus they all question the "central
alchemy" (Holton 1979) of the linear model.

But there are also differences among these critiques. Indeed, the rough
outlines of two broad camps can be discerned. Like the early bioethics of
the 1960s, a rich science policy initially reigned in conversations about

society-science relations that ranged widely across matters of purposes and ends (c.f., Dupree 1957; Snow 1959; Price 1965; Nelson 1968). In his conclusion, Daniel Greenberg (1968) exemplifies the substantive nature of this literature: "Finally, of infinitely greater importance than the bothersome book-keeping details that plague the relationship between science and government are the fundamental questions of purpose and value. What is it that man wants to do with his remarkable and growing power to investigate and manipulate the universe?" (Greenberg 1999, 292).

Beginning in the 1980s, however, this debate was replaced, with a few important exceptions,[7] by a much narrower focus. Wider considerations about the nature of the good life within a high-tech society and explicit discussions of values trade-offs faded out and were replaced by more instrumental rhetoric and practices for achieving predetermined goals. Chief among these, perhaps because it is often seen as a means to many goals, is the pursuit of economic growth via technological innovation. As Harvey Brooks explained, "[T]he end of the cold war brought a new surge of interest in tight social direction of science. This time, instead of reflecting goals of the Great Society, interest focused on international economic competition and private sector job creation" (Brooks 1996, 31). This instrumentalism—focused on how to transfer research to technology to productivity in the most efficient manner—is evident in much of the science and technology policy research throughout the 1980s and 1990s (c.f., Kuehn and Porter 1981;[8] Shapley and Roy 1985; Landau and Rosenberg 1986; Smith 1990; Kleinman 1995; Stokes 1997;[9] and Guston 2000[10]).

These developments in science policy research mirror science policy practice. The same decades witnessed strengthening ties between industry and government-funded research.[11] An increase in the ratio of private to public funding, combined with changing intellectual property regimes, strengthened linkages between private-sector priorities and publicly funded science. Booming economies in the developing world fueled worries about economic competitiveness. Corporate leaders and scientists presented their concerns in the National Academy of Sciences report, "Rising Above the Gathering Storm" (2005). This report articulates the tenet of instrumental science policy by arguing that economic growth is based largely on technological innovation and the equating of such growth with quality of life.[12]

In sum, questions of the ends of science and science policy have been largely displaced by a limited set of assumed ends. Science policy has become dominated by "economic reasoning," which "tends to shift discourse about science policy away from political questions of 'why?' and 'to what end?' to economic questions of 'how much?'" (Bozeman and Sarewitz 2005, 119). As we saw in part I, the questions about ends include considerations of which alternatives should be pursued, whether some lines of research or technological applications should be pursued at all, and what constitutes happiness in a high-tech society. Emphasizing the commercialization of research and technology does not resolve such questions, but rather replaces explicit consideration of them with an unconscious technological imperative. As just one example, biomedical innovation in the U.S. has advanced in parallel with increasing costs of health care and increasing disparities in access to health care both within the U.S. and between the developed and developing worlds (Callahan 1998). The default answer of innovation in the face of public health problems commits society to one determinant path among many, and in many cases it is not the optimal path.

In this and other contexts, ethics, science, and technology are inseparable. The question is whether or not the ethical dimensions of public decisions are recognized and debated reasonably and explicitly or channeled through default assumptions and motivating values. There is a need for a humanities policy to retrieve into reasonable and public forums of discussion a more explicit consideration of the ends of science and technology: innovation and growth for whom and to what end?

Humanities Policy: Beyond Instrumentalism

The upshot of my critique of policy instrumentalism has long been a theme for those who research the big picture of science policy: the "social contract" between society and science is in a crisis and in need of reform (e.g., Guston and Keniston 1994; Sonnert and Holton 2002). Most succinctly formulated by Bush in 1945, this contract presumes that the more the science, the more its (automatic) relevance and beneficence. But policy issues are value laden, and thus more than scientific or technical in character. And research almost always brings problems and challenges—"unintended consequences"—to accompany its benefits.[13]

Though many share in my analysis of the problem, few have examined the turn to humanistic inquiry as one possible solution (Briggle, Frodeman, and Holbrook 2006). Daniel Sarewitz (1996), for example, advances a lucid criticism of the linear model's social contract for science, but he stops short of prescribing a humanities policy. He argues that an emphasis on the outcomes of science policies requires assessment processes for judging the value of science and technology and guiding their development within a broader context of goods. He maintains that shifting "from the challenge of augmenting growth to the challenge of directing, responding to, and controlling it, ought to require as well a transition in the types of knowledge that humanity needs if it is to continue to move toward its most important goals" (Sarewitz 1996, 174). For Sarewitz, this knowledge can be found in the social sciences. It is "knowledge about how . . . progress occurs, how it can be directed in a matter most consistent with social and cultural norms and goals, and how it actually influences society" (174). He argues for "research that brings natural and social scientists together to focus on the creation of increased levels of compatibility between progress in the laboratory and social needs" (176). Sarewitz and David Guston have since implemented this important idea at the dynamic Consortium for Science, Policy, and Outcomes.

The social sciences, however, are themselves instrumental—capable of cataloguing values, but not assessing them.[14] Moral disagreement means that there is far more to do than simply match science more effectively to "social needs." What those needs should be and which ones ought to be met are precisely the questions at stake, and here the social sciences are mute. Addressing the ethical, political, theological, and aesthetic values driving science policy issues requires treating them not as irrational, but as amenable to reasonable discussion and re-formation through reflective, critical analysis. A humanistic reflection on ends can clarify, critique, and assess arguments and alternatives, rather than only measure preferences in hopes of more efficiently satisfying (some of) them.

Thus, implicit in humanities policy is a critique of the "social contract" metaphor that pictures politics as the practice of aggregating or trading preferences set antecedently in private by atomistic individuals, rather than mutually clarifying, transforming, and improving them.[15] As I argued in part I, the "contract" metaphor for our collective lives has always been a myth. In reality, we are not born with our "interests" set in advance. Rather, individuals develop values and commitments through fluid interactions with their changing societies. Only by focusing on short-term political cycles and the most extremely polarizing debates are we able to ignore the reality of society as a crucible in which meanings and values are formed and re-formed through human interactions.

Rich Humanities Policy

I hope to have established the need for a broader knowledge set—the humanities—in policy processes involving science and technology. This leaves open the more specific question of how the humanities can be relevant to policy. I suggested at the beginning of this chapter that there are two types of humanities policy. The distinction between them depends on how "policy" is conceptualized. The first, instrumentalist approach views policy as a sequence of isolated processes addressing specific issues in the short-term. The second, rich approach has a more holistic and substantive understanding of policy.

Bioethics advisory committees play a well-defined role within the first type of humanities policy. They formulate principles to guide action in a particular situation (e.g., research involving human subjects, cloning, or stem cell research), which entails advancing arguments and recommendations for and/or against competing alternatives in regard to a specific line of research, development, or application. The Kass Council played this role in nearly all of its reports, including recommendations and ethical analyses of policy alternatives about cloning, stem cell research, advance directives, and reproductive technologies. This sort of targeted, policy-specific assessment is presumably what the editors of *Nature Biotechnology* mean by "getting to the point," and indeed there is no doubting the value of such contributions by ethics committees.

What is less obvious, and therefore more in need of explicit defense, is the relevance of a rich humanities policy. Why, for example, would a federal advisory committee produce a report such as *Beyond Therapy* or—

with the Pellegrino Council—*Human Dignity and Bioethics,* which presents competing essays on the concept of dignity without producing a set of recommendations? Or to give the skeptic an even stronger case, of what possible policy relevance is an anthology of literature and poetry such as the Kass Council report *Being Human?* It is highly doubtful that policy makers will read such an anthology and directly apply it to a specific policy. If we take the instrumentalist approach to policy, then literature is irrelevant. But if we note that policy makers are products of their times that have stamped them with a certain way of being in and perceiving the world, then we can begin to understand how literature has policy relevance.

To see the relevance of *Being Human,* then, we need to see policy not as an isolated machine working only on the timelines of specific decisions and political cycles. Rather, we need to see the strands that connect this most visible aspect of policy to larger social and historical contexts. These more obvious parts of policy are the crests of waves jutting out from the moving, evolving ocean of human culture—both our material cultures of artifacts and systems and our ideational cultures of beliefs, values, and ideas. Indeed, we cannot isolate a purely instrumental policy process from these broader dimensions. For example, the Belmont principles of autonomy, beneficence, and justice are more than guidelines for human-subject research. They both reflect and reinforce important substantive ends in a liberal democracy founded on certain interpretations of justice, freedom, and individualism. The principles further articulate a deeply entrenched way of thinking and talking about being human. A different culture would produce a different policy.[16] This instrumentalist fix for a "policy vacuum," then, draws from and only makes sense in light of a wider frame of reference.

Alexis de Tocqueville characterized these wider horizons as "the slow and quiet action of society upon itself" (*Democracy in America* 1835, I, 18).[17] In a new media culture that consumes instantaneous news, it is easy to lose sight of the interplay of history and policy. Yet the connections are unbreakable. For example, the short policy cycles of civil rights legislation of the 1960s conditioned and were conditioned by more fundamental shifts in social values rooted in centuries of conflict. This example illustrates that—contrary to the assumptions of policy instrumentalism—the "issues" and "interests" involved in any given policy debate are not eternal, unchangeable givens that are already there. Policy is connected to a wider, multiperspectival public culture in which problems are not simply addressed but socially constructed, debated, and defined (Sabatier 1999).

Child labor in early industrial society is another case in point. Andrew Feenberg (1991) examines the debate surrounding the 1844 Factory Bill in England that eventually abolished child labor. The proposal was met with outrage by factory owners, who regarded child workers as an "imperative" of the system. They predicted dire inefficiencies and subsequent economic collapse if adult workers were required to replace children. At stake was not a simple policy issue, but a fundamental question about what a child is. Is a child a wage-laborer and a cog in the social means of production? This way of thinking about children had become prominent at the time. To counter this conception, a new mode of understanding children was needed. It was precisely this that Charles Dickens's popular 1830s magazine serial, then novel, *The Adventures of Oliver Twist* provided. Its vivid portrayals of poverty, cruelty, and misery made childhood imaginatively present and active within the adults of that age. The novel confronted them with the limits of the factory owners' way of thinking and stirred a sense of children as vulnerable, profound beings in need of love and protection.

The "environment" as an "issue" is another case where literature played a defining cultural role in elevating and transforming social consciousness to match the realities of the changing times. Advanced technological industrialism, as a new mode of human being-in-the-world, rests atop a certain way of understanding nature that Martin Heidegger (1954) called a "standing reserve," or nature understood as merely a collection of resources to be ordered and exploited. Poetic and literary works by John Muir, Henry David Thoreau, and others began to clear a space for alternative conceptions of nature. Aldo Leopold's *A Sand County Almanac* (1949) and Rachel Carson's *Silent Spring* (1962) further developed what would become "environmentalism." Though we will not be able to trace a direct "policy impact" of such works, it is hard to imagine a piece of legislation such as the 1964 Wilderness Act being achieved without their transformative effect on human thinking. Works of literature can in this way play an important role in shaping the foundations of awareness underlying a society's specific public policies.

So too with the current biomedical revolution, there is a need—in addition to reacting piecemeal to the countless policy decisions—to come to self-awareness of the changing times. Our ultimate course of action through the aggregate of laws and policies will depend on what we think it means to be human. It is at this deeper and slower layer of policy that *Being Human* finds relevance.

Literature and the Difficulty of Reality

I now return to the opening admonitions to "start with facts" and then "get to the point." Latent in such claims is an image, not only of public policy, but of moral philosophy as well. And it is an image, to borrow Heidegger's distinction, that may be correct but that is not altogether true. If we have only this conception of what it means to practice moral thought, then we will become like the drunk in the famous parable who is looking for his keys under the streetlamps because that is where it is easiest to see. I want to suggest that by its use of literature in *Being Human,* the Kass Council not only expanded its audience to classrooms but also extended its reach to other facets of popular culture. By bringing in literature, the council also invited its readers to practice a rich kind of moral inquiry, one that sees morality as continuous with our imaginative response to human life, including our capacity for sympathy (see Diamond 1991). In the growing use of literature and other humanities in bioethics classrooms, there is an emerging recognition of the importance of this kind of moral thinking (Chambers 1999; Charon and Montello 2005).

Instrumentalist moral thought is critiqued most cogently by Cora Diamond (1996), for whom instrumentalism takes moral thought to be the kind of thing that can occur only in arguments, just as it is commonly thought that mathematics occurs solely through proofs. We do not have *thought* unless we can rewrite the insight as argument. Poetry and other forms of art and literature may hint at ethical ideas, but they are not properly ethical until they have been abstracted out as issues to be examined. This is just another form of the isolationism intrinsic to instrumental thinking; isolate the "ethical issues" and treat them in a sequence of propositions and conclusions. Moral thought about a particular case consists in bringing rules and principles to bear on the *facts* of the case.

What is hidden here, as Diamond notes, is "the possibility that any moral thinking goes on in what one takes to be the facts of a case, how one comes to see them or describe them" (Diamond 1996, 310). There is something deeply problematic in taking "the facts" as simply given, because it perpetuates an unthinking recourse to the predominant moral resources at the shallow layer of policy discourse: are children best thought of as wage laborers, or nature as a bundle of resources? Similarly, for biotechnology policy the "factual" question "what is it to be human?" has deeply moral dimensions that literature can illuminate.

In all these cases, the deeper layer of public policy lies closer to intuitions, which are, for the time being, considered foreign or illegitimate in the debates at the shallow level. There is, then, a tension inherent in their relationship. In order to correct for the distortions and narrowness that inevitably encrust the shallow layer, there needs to be an upsurge from below that works to transform thought and refresh our moral language and vision (see May 2005).

It is here that a rich moral philosophy of literature becomes relevant in helping us to recognize and see beyond the limits of understanding within ethics-as-argumentation. Literature is not simply ideas and arguments concealed in fictional form. It is not an obstacle to our attempts to correspond with "the facts" of the world. Indeed, as Heidegger (1954) notes, the root meaning of truth is not correspondence between a proposition and an external state of affairs. Rather, truth or *alethia* is a revealing or a bringing forth out of concealment: "a" is the Greek privative, denoting an absence, and "lethe" means forgetfulness or slumber (cf. the river Lethe). *Alethia,* then, means an understanding of truth as an unforgetting or un-concealing; put differently, "truthing" occurs when we realize something, that is, when it becomes richly meaningful to us. This is the sort of truth offered by good literature that is read with care.

Diamond notes that the link "between the task of the literary artist and the ethical task is implicitly denied when moral thought is limited to the direction of choice between fixed and readily grasped possibilities, with the idea that it is not for us as moral agents to struggle to make sense of things" (Diamond 1996, 312). Narrative fiction is a distinctive epistemology that is true to our lives as ethical, biographical agents constantly struggling to interpret the world as we enact our own stories. Through great literature, the mysteries of existence shine through the carefully wrought fabric of human stories. Further, through literature we come to "see ourselves" in different scenarios, thus educating our characters by enhancing our moral sympathy and imagination.[18]

Diamond (2006) summarizes the task of a rich moral philosophy as "the difficulty of attempting to bring a difficulty of reality into focus." *Being Human* sets out to further our understanding of what it means to be human. It uses literature because this is a mode of understanding that can capture the difficult reality of being human—the difficulty of matching thought to our complex, often contradictory beings. The difficulty is the resistance of reality to our ordinary modes of living and thinking. To appreciate reality is to become "shouldered out" of one's common way of thinking or sense of how one is supposed to think. It is to have a feeling for the inability of thought to encompass what it is trying to reach. It is this difficulty that is "deflected" and presented only in a diminished and distorted way in philosophical argumentation. Furthermore, in ordinary life and with the ordinary concepts used at the shallow level of policy, we pass by the difficulty as if it were not there. But a poem by Galway Kinnell (1980), for example, awakens the reader to the difficult mystery of being mortal, being creatures of love, and of generational bonds. A father speaking of his son in "After Making Love We Hear Footsteps" reflects,

> this one whom habit of memory propels to the ground of his making,
> sleeper only the mortal sounds can sing awake,
> this blessing love gives again into our arms.

What Good Are the Humanities?

Stanley Fish (2008) concluded his *New York Times* op-ed piece "Will the Humanities Save Us?" by arguing that the humanities "don't do anything, if by 'do' is meant bring about effects in the world." It is the old *l'art pour l'art* justification: "The humanities are their own good, there is nothing more to say." And indeed, this is an alluring image of the humanities at a time when the pressures of the entrepreneurial, science- and technology-driven university are increasing the demand for practical (that is, economically demonstrable) results. What could be more radical than simply following the native progression of thought in homage to "irrelevance," thereby implicitly indicting the modern obsession with utility?

To the contrary, I have argued that the humanities are relevant to public policy. But such relevance cannot be framed as knowledge being "useful" for satisfying needs or accomplishing goals. It is true that relevance is often interpreted in instrumental terms in light of given, short-range goals. Yet, I have used *Being Human* as an occasion for thinking about an alternative sense of relevance. Often what is most needed in a society jaded by the "progress paradox" is an enriched reflection on the worthiness of the goals society sets for us and their relation to meaningful lives. As the Cistercian monk Thomas Merton noted, "modern man" does not understand "that, at bottom, it is the useful that may be a useless . . . burden" (Merton 1964, 21). I would only add the converse point that the apparently useless may be of the greatest importance. Relevance may be necessarily goal-dependent (something can only be relevant *to* or *for* a given purpose), but these goals need not be cast solely as utilitarian, immediate, or material in nature. And they must not be cast as unproblematic—it is often most relevant to ask how an "issue" ought to be framed, which in the context of biomedical science and technology policy often necessitates a deeper and wider perspective on the difficulty of being human.

Conclusion

Public Philosophy in a Liberal Democracy

In book VI of *The Republic*, Socrates compares the state to a ship and reflects on the nature of a good captain. "The true pilot," he argues, "must give his attention to the time of the year, the seasons, the sky, the winds, the stars, and all that pertains to his art if he is to be a true ruler of a ship." Similarly, to navigate the ship of state well requires the union of authority with the steerer's art. Socrates makes it clear that this art — the requisite skill for true political leadership — is philosophy. In the activity of stargazing, he finds an apt metaphor for the philosopher's grasp of the eternal and unchangeable. All nonphilosophers are lost and "wander in the region of the many and variable." The nonphilosophic crew of the ship "does not understand that the art of navigation demands knowledge of the stars." Therefore they will stigmatize the true pilot "as a stargazer, an idle babbler, a useless fellow" and prevent him from navigating (see *Republic* VI, 488–90). This is why actual societies fall short of the ideal.

The ideal city should be ruled by philosopher kings, because only they have knowledge of the Good, and thus only they can steer the ship of state toward its attainment. However ideal Socrates' parable may be in theory, in practice it is disastrous. At the heart of Plato's vision is not only a very un-Kantian elitism—only a few can know enough about the Good to make informed decisions about it—but also *monism:* there is one best way to live. Isaiah Berlin (1998) traces this idea through history, arguing that it is responsible for countless depredations of tyrants seeking to forcibly impose their vision of the Good on the benighted masses. Berlin counters Plato with an alternative ideal, which he calls *pluralism.* In the eighteenth century, Giambattista Vico and Johann Herder began to envision politics as the association of different, perhaps even equally valid conceptions of how to live.

Such defenses of pluralism became wedded to the solution proffered by Hobbes and Locke to the religious wars of their time: relegate conflicting conceptions of the good to the private sphere. The modern liberal self is a sovereign bearer of rights and author of obligations and ends. If ultimate questions of meaning and flourishing are personal affairs, confined to this atomistic subject, then government is restricted to matters of the right. Moral pluralism would thereby be protected from the coercive imposition of a monistic doctrine of the good. As Kass Council member Michael Sandel put it, "statecraft no longer needs soulcraft" (Sandel 1996, 70). The privatization of ends or personal "life plans" would spare politics the ancient quarrels about the nature of the good life.

Berlin, Robert Dahl (1998), and others are in one sense justifiably skittish about the mix of democracy and philosophy. Of course, in a world dependent on technology, it is increasingly the case that democracy "is a form of collaboration of ignorant people and experts" (Schattschneider 1960, 137). But when those experts are doing ethics, many see foreboding intimations of Plato's "ideal" city displacing even the core instances of popular sovereignty remaining in a modern bureaucratic nation state. Ethics experts might command the moral authority to dictate public policy and overrule personal choice.

Yet in many ways, such fears are unfounded, as over the course of the twentieth century philosophers have largely adopted the disciplinary model of knowledge production. They have thus taken leave of the city to sequester themselves in the ivory towers (Kucklick 1977). When they returned to the city in 1974, with theologians and other humanists, to sit on bioethics commissions, they were hardly crowned as kings.[1] Indeed, their powers over governmental affairs were immensely more limited and less grand than captains of the ship of state. They were, in short, philosopher bureaucrats, not kings (Frodeman 2006).

In a liberal democracy, philosophic expertise derives its epistemological warrant not from the truth of one's judgments but from the ability of the expert to provide reasonable and persuasive justification for his or her claims (Walzer 1981; Brock 1987; Yoder 1998; Johnson 2007). The task of rich public bioethics is to make and evaluate representations that stand for diverse positions, but not to make ultimate decisions in the form of policies. It is to enable citizens to understand and challenge such public decisions (see Brown 2008). Furthermore, in the context of federal ethics advisory bodies, ethical elitism—the usurpation of power by the wise few—is not even a viable concern. For example, while the Belmont Report has had perhaps greater impact on governance than any other report by a bioethics commission, in no sense was it an edict imposed from on high by wise kings. Like all federal advice, it had to wend its way through the sausage factory of policy making with all of its political checks and balances. Indeed, if anything, expert knowledge, whether scientific or philosophic, has in contemporary politics too little influence. Advisory bodies and other intelligence-producing agencies are routinely ignored or used as mere fodder in partisan games (Hudson 2004; Pielke 2007).

We are in this sense a long way from philosopher kings. Nonetheless, bioethics commissions prior to the Kass Council severely limited the scope of their moral inquiry. They largely restricted their considerations to matters of the right, presuming to leave questions of the good to personal inclination. As Evans (2002) notes, this was the result of a jurisdictional battle which the new discipline of bioethics, along with scientific and medical researchers, won. Instrumentalism has been justified, however, not as the result of a turf war, but as a necessary result of two theses. The first is the privatization thesis, which holds that matters of the good are in point of fact personal decisions. They thus occur solely in the private sphere, and government can and should provide a neutral framework within which each citizen can pursue the good as he or she understands it. The second thesis holds that these decisions are fundamentally irrational, because choices about good lives are expressions of subjective wants and not, contra Plato and Kant, amenable to improvement through processes of reasoned inquiry.

If both theses (privatization and irrationality) are true, then we must follow Hobbes and Engelhardt (1996) down the social contract path and conclude that the only necessary and legitimate form of public philosophy in a pluralist society is instrumentalism. This is so, according to this argument, because legitimacy can be grounded either in citizenship, in which everyone is entitled to their opinion, or in specialized means-ends knowledge, such as that found in science, engineering, or instrumental bioethics. An "ends commission" cannot have any legitimacy beyond that of the average "man on the street." According to this view, "If you take democracy seriously, then the basic rule is that every philosopher is simply a citizen, and every citizen a philosopher, capable of making decisions that reflect his or her conscientiously held beliefs" (Shalit 1997, 347). The implication is that publicly sponsored philosophic inquiry into questions of what constitutes good lives is both a waste of resources (because there is no knowledge or improved understanding to be found) and a threat to pluralism (because philosophic ethics presumes there is one right answer).

With these two theses we have arrived at the very opposite position from that of Plato's philosopher kings. There is now no room for philosophy—understood as knowledge of ends or the good—at all, certainly not philosophic ethics as part of government. Evans makes this plain when he substitutes social science for ethics and argues that public bioethics should focus on developing "a more accurate process of measuring the values of the public" and that "social science has the ability to do this measurement" through "survey and interview methodologies" (Evans 2006, 229). For Evans, like Philip Kitcher (2001),[2] expertise is only instrumental. Thus public "philosophers" are reduced to measuring—not evaluating— values.

Evans argues that the instrumentalism practiced by bioethics committees prior to the Kass Council was pernicious because its "technocratic" approach means that "expert rule is justified by making policy decisions *seem to be* only about facts . . . and not about values" (Evans 2006, 217). The principles of autonomy, safety, and justice are presented as if they are the goals, as a matter of fact, accepted by society without open debate, and that the remaining work is finding out how to achieve and balance them. In proposing his model, Evans overturns this elitism by requiring that public philosophy be justified by the standards of the public sphere rather than those of professionals. This is all well and good. Yet Evans retains the thesis that the standards of the public sphere are essentially personal preferences, among which there is no reasonable way of determining better and worse. The Kass Council, so I have argued, modeled an alterative to this skepticism by fostering reasonable inquiry into goods, or as its mandate phrased the matter, the human significance of biomedical science and technology.

Statecraft and Soulcraft: A Perfectionist Model of Public Philosophy

The reason for my defense of a rich bioethics is that the two theses (privatization and irrationality) do not hold. First, I have demonstrated that matters of the good cannot be confined to the private sphere; we can only pretend to do so while working with unarticulated, default substantive visions in our collective affairs. Government constantly shapes the life-world, creating conditions that promote some ways of life and discourage others. This is particularly true with the regulation and promotion of science and technology. To sustain a rich forum of public moral debate is not to violate an alleged neutrality of the good, but rather to explicitly recognize and discuss what had previously been cast in shadow. The purpose of such discussions is to foster improved understanding about human flourishing and its relation to biomedical science and technology.

Second, the rich bioethics model supports the view that such improved understanding can be achieved. Values pluralism, as Berlin argued, is not the same as ethical subjectivism. Certainly basic values do come into conflict and reasonable people may disagree on how to rank their importance. Nonetheless, communication and understanding of moral views is possible, because the values we pursue are rooted in our common—though variable and complex—human nature. It is this nature that makes autonomy, the freedom to choose one's own path, good and desirable for human beings. Indeed, liberalism's commitment to pluralism and the freedom to change one's mind is premised on the ideal that we can make changes for the better by openly and freely engaging with other perspectives. Both subjectivism and monism are too rigid to do justice to our capacity for moral development and improved moral insight through conversation.

It is the failure of the two instrumentalist theses that opens up both the need for and the possibility of a rich public inquiry into human goods. In both our personal and public deliberations and decisions about biomedical science and technology, we confront questions about the meaning of living well. The promise of a rich public moral inquiry is that we can approach these questions more self-consciously and collaboratively.

The threats of Plato's model of public philosophy are clear, but consider the absurdity of its opposite as espoused by Evans (2006). He leaves us either with the mere measuring of preferences or with a Madisonian model of public philosophy. Public philosophers serve as the house intellectuals for different interest groups. There would be Republican and Democratic philosophers, right-to-life and pro-choice philosophers, philosophers for the posthumanists and the Luddites, etc. Such "public philosophers" are neither philosophers (because they only espouse foregone conclusions) nor public (because they take only one special interest standpoint). They are, as Socrates might note, mere sophists.

What society needs and what the Kass Council modeled, albeit imperfectly, is a middle way capable of protecting what is true and important about liberalism from the excesses of both elitist monism and subjectivism. Contemporary society tends not to see that subjectivism is coercive in its own right. It licenses without critical reflection implicit conceptions of the good worked out mainly through a consumerist technological imperative. The tyranny we face is less that of philosopher kings than that of unreflective preferences deformed by a narrow utilitarian habit of mind and multiplied infinitely by a consumer economy that increasingly pictures the human condition as a series of problems to be solved with the latest technological breakthrough. The danger is that we will lose sight of what is humanly meaningful and important amidst all the bluster of what is technically possible. The peril is that despite "progress" we will languish, exhausted on a hedonic treadmill, rather than flourish both as a society and as individuals, because we did not pause to critically evaluate our desires.

Seen in this light, the Kass Council's rich public bioethics was a novel institutional expression of liberal perfectionism.[3] This political theory holds that it is "legitimate for the government (a) to promote the ethical flourishing of its citizens, while (b) relying on a more-than-want-regarding notion of what such flourishing consists in" (Appiah 2005, 157). In other words, it is a position that denies both that the good can be confined to the private sphere and that the good is simply a matter of subjective preferences. Appiah observes that "there has never been a state without some influence upon the character of its citizens" (Appiah 2005, 155). Thus, statecraft cannot actually be practiced without soulcraft; the practice can be only more or less explicitly recognized and debated.

The question is how much and in what ways the state should encourage the ethical flourishing of its citizens. Following a similar "pluralist perfectionist" theory, council member Robert George (1993) argues that "moral laws" aimed at preserving the moral ecology of a society can play a legitimate, albeit subsidiary, role in liberal societies. This may in fact be the case, but my argument for the Kass Council is less controversial, because it was not authorized to craft regulatory or otherwise coercive legislation. Indeed, this would be a wholly inappropriate role for a group of unelected professionals. The council did not even have the power to enforce existing legislation. It was to be a public forum of advice and deliberation.

Rather than morals legislation, the model of perfectionism most like the Kass Council is liberal education. Indeed, it is helpful to think of rich public philosophy as a kind of state-sponsored education in addition to the traditional role of policy advice. Here, the government promotes ethical flourishing by encouraging its citizens to become more educated about the decisions they face and the desires they hold. Bioethics commissions are ideal places for this kind of liberal perfectionism, because they have no legislative authority, command wide audiences, and have the prestige to bring together leading thinkers from all perspectives into conversation with one another. It is interesting here to note Kass's own insight on this score: "In liberal democracy, and especially in liberal education, lies the last best hope of mankind" (Kass 2002, 52). Of course, liberal democracy is only the last best hope if it is conceived of as a counterweight to, rather than an extension of, the market. It is only something hopeful if it is a public arena in which we reflect on and improve our desires rather than merely express them.

Conversation

What we discover when we leave the cave of our local conventions is a stunning diversity of ways of life. This prompts the first question of ethics:

Given all of these possible answers to the human condition, how should I live? Only once we have removed blind allegiance to the authority of convention can we practice that philosophical wonder behind questions about the meaning of human existence.

With the blinders of convention removed, we are in a sense liberated, but the freedom we have is not of the boundless existentialist variety. Rather, our freedom is an interpretive response to encountered circumstances, most of which we did not create. If we are not to feel imprisoned or paralyzed by chaos, we will require social institutions and capable teachers to initiate us into and make sense of the world we inhabit. Such structures issue what Michael Oakeshott calls "the invitation of liberal learning," which is an invitation "to listen to the conversation in which human beings forever seek to understand themselves" (Oakeshott 1989, 41).

As an ideal, rich public bioethics shares with liberal learning this same simple essence of the conversation. It is commonplace to lament the declining art of conversation in times of unprecedented polarization and a new media age that seems paradoxically to produce both enormous channels for information exchange and a general decline in the quality of communication (e.g., Sunstein 2007). Many follow Englehardt (1996) in presuming that there are irreducible barriers that restrict moral communication to only the thinnest of principles.

But as Walter Lippmann (1955) noted in his own call to revive a "public philosophy," such stories too easily become fatalistic, as if it were not within our power to recover a more civil and refined public dialogue about the challenges we face in common. It is true that even as modernity works to bind our collective fate ever more tightly, it scatters and dissolves traditional communities of discourse. Nonetheless, we can compensate for this dissolution. It is more productive to pay attention to those instances in public life—such as bioethics commissions—where we can listen in on and participate in conversations that cross boundaries in the examination of our common humanity.

A conversation is a discussion conducted by people practicing mutual tolerance for opposing viewpoints (Miller 2007). Instrumentalist bioethics sustains conversation, but only in the limited sense of an exchange of ideas about how best to achieve or balance a given set of goods. Biomedical science and technology call for an enlarged conversation to make us more self-conscious and to criticize the range of goods at stake and the

competing evaluations proffered by the diverse voices comprising a pluralist moral community.

This task calls for what Plato in the *Statesman* considered the highest
form of knowledge: dialectics or conversation, which brings out of concealment the "what is" of things. This also saves us from a simplistic understanding of Plato's notion of public philosophy. After all, in the opening scene of *The Republic,* Plato depicts philosophy as an alternative to
coercion that casts doubt on the notion of a philosopher as a ruling king.
Socrates understood that philosophy cannot be a solitary affair. Due to the
weakness of individual minds, genuine knowledge must be intersubjec-
tive in nature.[4] Philosophy necessarily leads to skepticism about all human
claims to understanding, including the philosopher's own claims. In the
Lysis, Socrates' teaching about philosophy is essentially a teaching about
friendship—philosophy is the patient and dynamic pursuit of wisdom
amongst friends who are not yet, and most likely never will be, wise.

But friendship, if it is not open and cosmopolitan, creates outsiders
who do not share the same opinions and practices, and thus there is a
danger that philosophers may devolve into sects or interest groups. This
is another way to see the criticisms that many had of the Kass Council—
it was, they claim, a stealth ideology advocate for a single doctrine of the
good, not a broker of a friendly conversation among diverse traditions.[5] I
have argued that there were some good reasons for thinking this in light
of certain practices that point toward the need for changes in future public bioethics. But in general, the accusation does not hold under a fair reading of the Kass Council's reports. Its work sometimes advanced deeply
divergent recommendations and at other times it made conclusions in
line with a particular view of the good life. But in these cases it often did so
by fostering a conversation and an exchange of arguments between competing substantive positions on issues from cloning and reprogenetics to
caring for the aging and physical and mental enhancements. This is far
more conducive to the kind of pluralist conversation that we need than
the instrumentalist tactic of dismissing such matters from the start as off
limits. Again, our choice is how to handle such substantive issues, explicitly or implicitly, not whether to handle them.

Nonetheless, the critics of the Kass Council highlight the crucial point:
a rich conversation must work to cross boundaries of difference. Such an
image of conversation comes from the Hebrew scriptures, where it implies

less an act of verbal communication than a relationship of citizens within a community. It thus replaces an image of autonomous selves engaged in contracts to fulfill their unchangeable preferences, with a communal image of the self as continuously shaped by human interactions. Mutual respect and understanding are fostered by "conversation—not mere debate but the disciplined act of communicating (making my views intelligible to someone who does not share them) and listening (entering into the inner world of someone whose views are opposed to my own) . . . a sustained act of understanding and seeking to be understood across the boundaries of difference" (Sacks 2003, 83).

Contemporary ethical debate often involves several traditions, or systems of belief, with divergent first principles. For a substantive conversation, what is required of an individual confronting the competing claims of rival traditions is to learn "how to test dialectically the theses proposed to him or her by each competing tradition, while also drawing upon these same theses in order to test dialectically those convictions and responses which he or she has brought to the encounter. Such a person has to become involved in the conversation between traditions, learning to use the idiom of each in order to describe and evaluate the other or others by means of it" (MacIntyre 1988, 398).

Ethical pluralism calls us to seek out truths in others' views and modify our own. It involves "acknowledging that different ways of life and conceptions of human good are not necessarily closed and incomplete but can be receptive to elements found in other ways of life and conceptions of the good" (Cohen 2005b, 285).

Because the bar is set pretty low, contemporary U.S. society is bound to continue the permissive, if not enthusiastic, political strategies that have given rise to our present technological condition. As long as a technology is not unduly harmful (and in many cases even this does not seem to matter), it can be sent to the market where individuals can decide (within the constraints noted in chapter 3) whether or not to adopt it. Bans may have some selective role to play, and indeed the council debated them along with other forms of regulation. But bans and government regulation more generally are limited in both principle and practice. New technologies will enter the market. The question then becomes a matter of individual choice. This is why we need to consider not just the scope of such choice, but also the kind or quality of awareness with which people work out their lives.

I have argued that a rich kind of thinking and conversing is needed if we are to improve our quality of awareness—our wisdom—and thus our ability to shape technology for a better future. Nietzsche saw this at a time when modern technology was just beginning to fulfill its promise of lightening the burden of human existence: "There are some who threw away their last value when they threw away their servitude. Free *from* what? As if that mattered to Zarathustra! But your eyes should tell me brightly: free *for* what?" That is the question that rich bioethics poses—what is the vision of progress and a better humanity that is driving our unprecedented investments in biotechnology? Is it a worthy vision?

The benefits of a rich conversation around this question will not likely come in the form of immediate policy "impacts," just as liberal education or *Bildung* is not vocational training. Through the critical examination of one's own and others' moral positions, the real fruits of conversation will come at deeper cultural and personal levels. One way to understand the benefits of rich bioethics is in terms of a theory of "informed desire satisfaction." One will get a better sense of what truly is desirable by becoming aware of the consequences of all the different choices available as they are made real through imagination and argument. A person may come, for example, to doubt the value of a life that includes the use of pharmacological enhancements—a life that at first glance seemed immensely attractive. In this way, she may come to reconsider and revise her values and life plans in response to fresh insights and an expanded imagination. Since the whole point is about human well-being, we need to be thoughtful about what it means to flourish. We need guidance on what constitutes a worthy choice, not just procedures for protecting free, safe, and fair choices.

The transformation of bare to informed preferences is a reasonable way to consider the value of rich public bioethics conversation. And it is compatible with the perfectionist ideal of, in Berlin's terms, "positive liberty" or the idea that in certain ways humans require help from the state and from fellow citizens to achieve their better selves. We owe it to one another, as Mill argued, to help distinguish the better from the worse.

But even if we have a reasonable definition of what it would mean to possess "adequately informed" desires, I do not think it is best to conceive of the fruits of rich conversation in terms of subjective preferences. This is because subjectivism, as a stand-alone theory, is a severely flawed account of human flourishing, and its flaws are not removed by substituting informed for bare preferences. The subjectivist desire-satisfaction theory holds that something is valuable just in case, and because, it would contribute to the satisfaction of desires. But as David Brink notes, "this seems to get things just about the opposite way around in many cases; we desire certain sorts of things *because we think these things valuable*" (Brink 1989, 225). Indeed, many of the activities, traits, and relationships that we intuitively consider part of a meaningful and worthy life (e.g., autonomy, knowledge, excellence, friendship, and virtue) often do not satisfy the desires of their possessors.

The question that a rich conversation helps us face is not which alternative we *do* most want (if we had informed desires), but rather which alternative is most *worth* wanting: "to find out, we try to look *past* our current desires and preferences to the value or disvalue of the objects" (Sher 1997, 186). This kind of questioning is commonplace to our decision making, as we regularly presuppose that we are responding to values that exist prior to our desires or choices and thus that some things are more worthy of choice than others. What rich public bioethics provides, in both its substance and holism, is help as we engage in these decisions. Aristotle sums this up:

> For each man has something of his own to contribute to the finding of the truth, and it is from such (starting points) that we must demonstrate: beginning with things that are correctly said, but not clearly, as we proceed we shall come to express them clearly, with what is more perspicuous at each stage superseding what is customarily expressed in a confused fashion . . . So the political man, also, should not regard as irrelevant not only the *that* but also the *why*. For that way of proceeding is the philosopher's. (*Eudemian Ethics,* 1216b26–40)

Aristotle suggests a public philosopher who begins with a plurality of views and then, with patience and an open mind, sifts through them in hopes of transforming what was muddled into something more intelligible. In so doing, he paints a picture of pluralism neither as the expression of millions of irreducibly incommensurable viewpoints nor as an indication that all but a few of us have arrived at the wrong conclusion. Rather, pluralism is an opportunity. It is the chance to refine our own perspective and expand our moral outlook. It offers the prospect of charting a course through triangulation. In this way, a rich public philosophy helps us become more clear-eyed as we navigate both the ship of state and our personal lives through waters made turbulent by scientific and technological change.

NOTES

Introduction

1. The executive order expired after two years, but the council was renewed by President Bush by means of Executive Order 13316 on September 23, 2003. Of his own initiative, Kass stepped down as chair just prior to the second of such renewals (Executive Order 13385, September 29, 2005). Dr. Edmund Pellegrino took over as chair, and Kass remained on the Pellegrino Council as a regular member for most of its existence. The Pellegrino Council continued to operate throughout the Bush presidency. For the most part, it receded from the spotlight of American politics and slowed its productivity, producing only one report in three years.

2. Throughout this book the terms "council" and "Kass Council" will be used interchangeably to refer to the council under the chairmanship of Kass.

3. Some commentators on bioethics commissions would parse these two tasks as "expertise" and "agenda-setting." The former denotes the provision of specialized knowledge for policymaking, whereas the latter denotes public engagement and deliberation and the elevation of public understanding (see Dzur and Levin 2004).

4. All minutes for the meetings of the Kass Council are available on the council's Web site, at http://www.bioethics.gov.

ONE   Public Bioethics and the Birth of the Kass Council

1. For an overview of the historical rise of the concept of autonomy in Western moral philosophy, see Schneewind 1998.

2. Of the twenty-three defendants, five were acquitted, and seven received death sentences; the remaining received prison sentences ranging from ten years to life imprisonment. Japan also engaged in large-scale medical experiments during World War II that included similar atrocious acts. The experiments were primarily conducted on Chinese citizens. Japanese research was never subjected to judicial scrutiny (Rothman 2004).

3. In 1930, the Berlin Medical Board proposed a regulatory body to review human-subjects research, which precipitated a debate about the ethics of clinical drug trials within the context of an increasingly powerful German pharmaceuti-

cal industry. A set of guidelines released in 1931, the legal authority of which was contested, was more comprehensive and cogent than the Nuremberg Code (see Howard-Jones 1982).

4. This is not to claim that a basic respect for persons was absent from pre-modern ethical thought on human experimentation. For example, in the twelfth century, Moses Maimonides instructed colleagues to treat patients as ends in themselves, not as means for learning new truths (see Rothman 2004).

5. The committee was called the Seattle Artificial Kidney Center's Admission and Policy Committee.

6. Cases such as this eventually led to the Baby Doe regulations of 1984, which state that withholding neonatal intensive care on the basis of handicap (or in the case of extremely premature infants, increased risk of handicap) was deemed to be discrimination and a violation of the Rehabilitation Act of 1973.

7. Of course, medical codes of ethics had long existed (e.g., the 1847 American Medical Association code). Such codes primarily addressed patient-physician relations. But it was not until the 1970s that formal regulations on biomedical research were implemented. These were novel in being government-mandated rules rather than professional self-regulations and in focusing on research rather than medical practice (though the boundary between the two is blurry—clinical practice often contributes to scientific knowledge, and research trials are often administered by physicians and have therapeutic effects).

8. Beecher's work demonstrates that some of the impetus for external oversight came from within the scientific and medical communities. This parallels the "responsible science movement" of the 1950s, in which scientists and engineers sought to control the direction of science and technology in light of the destructive potential of atomic weapons.

9. In the mid-twentieth century, the U.S. government also conducted radiation experiments on U.S. citizens who were not fully informed about the health risks; however, these experiments were not revealed until the 1990s and so did not influence the prehistory of U.S. public bioethics. The unethical treatment of human subjects is a continuing problem. For example, accusations arose in early 2005 that U.S. physicians cooperated in the torture of prisoners at the Abu Ghraib prison in Iraq.

10. Indeed, bioethics grew out of medical ethics: "If traditional medical ethics was a form of self-critique and self-control, bioethics, at least initially, represented public critique and public control" (Dzur and Levin 2004, 336).

11. This is in contrast to more specific bodies such as institutional review boards, institutional biosafety committees, and the Recombinant DNA Advisory Committee, which have responsibility for reviewing, approving, regulating, or overseeing specific projects or government agencies.

12. Interestingly, this is also the case for National Ethics Councils in Western Europe, but increasingly such Councils in Eastern Europe are mandated to form legislation (see Ahvenharju et al. 2006).

13. In 1954, Joseph Murray performed the first successful kidney transplant, but subsequent developments in immunosuppressive drugs and the invention of the heart-lung machine led to greater success in organ transplantation beginning in the late 1960s.

14. The recommendations were made by an NIH advisory panel, the Human Embryology and Development Study Section.

15. The phrase "public bioethics" was coined by John Fletcher (1994) to denote "inquiry supported by government to identify the major ethical considerations and public policy implications of controversial issues in biomedicine" (184). I use bioethics committees or commissions as synonyms for public bioethics institutions.

16. One interesting note is that Congress included a "forcing" clause in the legislation that created the National Commission. The clause required the Secretary of DHEW to accept recommendations within 180 days or publish reasons for not accepting them in the *Federal Register.*

17. As noted above, IRBs had existed since 1966, but it was only at this time that they became a mandatory part of NIH funded research (Fletcher and Miller 1996).

18. This dominance can be seen by looking at the table of contents of other influential textbooks. Veatch (2003) discusses only traditional ethical topics, except for some consideration of issues concerning human nature. Mappes and Degrazia (2001) devote just one chapter late in the book to matters of genetics and human nature. Glannon (2005) and Beauchamp and Walters (2003) feature a similar taxonomy. Holland (2003) discusses the idea of the "natural" as a normative concept. Yet he dismisses normative appeals to the natural as either bad ethics or a psychological coping mechanism. This text, like the majority of bioethics textbooks, does not stray far from the framework of principlism.

19. The U.S. had an effective moratorium on the federal funding of IVF research since 1975, although privately funded research was being performed.

20. The appointment of the chair was subject to Senate confirmation.

21. The twelve member panel was evenly bipartisan. This was modeled on the Technology Assessment Board, which oversaw the Office of Technology Assessment.

22. One example is the President's Council's recommendation to increase the use of living wills and the Kass Council's criticism of an over-reliance on living wills.

23. The OTA report recognized trade-offs between a distributed network of topical initiatives and a centralized commission. But it is not a zero-sum game; the creation of a national commission does not stop the decentralized network of institutions from operating.

24. The committee's work later led to the book by its senior staff member Jonathan Moreno, *Undue Risk: Secret State Experiments on Humans* (1999). The

committee was a response in part to a 1986 report by the staff of Massachusetts Congressman Ed Markey, *American Nuclear Guinea Pigs.*

25. Another cloning report was produced in 2002 by the National Academy of Sciences (NAS). Dolly was born in July 1996, but her birth was not made public by the Roslin Institute until February 1997.

26. This law does not address the private sector. It is about what taxpayers can support rather than what is legal.

27. The scientists were working with private money from the Geron Corporation and the University of Wisconsin Alumni Research Foundation.

28. The Senate, however, remained stalled on a related bill, largely due to different opinions about cloning for biomedical research and cloning to produce children. Thus no ban was enacted.

29. The policy allows federal funding only on stem cell lines that existed prior to August 9, 2001

30. This information was obtained via e-mail correspondence with Diane Gianelli, director of communication, Kass Council staff, on October 15, 2004.

31. For similar analyses, see Pellegrino (1999) and Moreno (2005).

32. Other examples of this thicker debate can be seen in historian Donald Fleming's article "On Living in a Biological Revolution" (1969) and Gordon Taylor's *Biological Time Bomb* (1968).

33. This is also true of national ethics councils (NECs) within Europe, where principlism has dominated for roughly the past two decades. A report commissioned by the European Commission notes that principlism "has been the dominant approach" taken by NECs and that many of the reports "follow the principlist approach quite literally" by dividing their analyses into parts corresponding to the principles of respect for autonomy, nonmaleficence, beneficence, and justice (Ahvenharju et al. 2006, 35).

34. The report by Sanna Ahvenharju et al. (2006) makes a similar point. They argue that the work of the European NECs becomes problematic when multidimensional issues are reduced to more simplistic framings. This is precisely one of the major problems with instrumentalism: in reducing complex bioethical quandaries to a very narrow set of principles and means-ends reasoning, it obscures or even prohibits an ethical analysis that can be adequate to the many dimensions of such issues.

35. This is another way to frame the importance of the Kass Council's commitment to being a council on bioethics (as an interdisciplinary conversation) rather than a council of bioethicists (as a narrow expert group with specific methods and commitments).

36. In the executive summary of *Human Cloning and Human Dignity,* the council provides its own justification for this approach: "On some matters discussed in this report, Members of the council are not of one mind. Rather than bury these differences in search of a spurious consensus, we have sought to present

all views fully and fairly, while recording our agreements as well as our genuine diversity of perspectives, including our differences on the final recommendations to be made. By this means, we hope to help policymakers and the general public appreciate more thoroughly the difficulty of the issues and the competing goods that are at stake" (Kass Council 2002, xxiii).

TWO   **The Deeper History of the Kass Council**

1. Though its roots do indeed reach into deep historical soil, the actual word "bioethics" is of very recent coinage. It has two origins. First, biologist Van Renesselar Potter (1971) defined "bioethics" as a naturalistic ethics based on biological science. Second, in the early 1970s, Andre Hellegers and others at the Kennedy Institute coined the term "bioethics" to denote the application of ethical theories or principles to dilemmas raised by biomedicine. The term entered the Library of Congress catalogue as a subject head in 1974, citing Callahan's 1973 essay "Bioethics as a Discipline" as its authority. The first bioethics course was taught in 1974 at the University of Tennessee, and in 1976 a Ph.D. program with a concentration in bioethics began at Georgetown University. For a detailed historical and sociological account of bioethics in America see Renèe Fox and Judith Swazey 2008.

2. Of course, Aristotle and Plato often differed on major points. Plato's work is erotic and takes the form of narrative, while Aristotle's thought is crisply analytical. Perhaps most importantly for this survey, Aristotle allowed for a much greater heterogeneity of goods and for uncertainty in ethical knowledge, whereas Plato tended to be more homogenous in seeking the one true good. For Aristotle, all natural right is changeable in a way that it is not for Plato. Strauss (1953) interprets Aristotle as meaning that there is a universally valid hierarchy of ends, but no generalizable set of rules for determining them. Context always matters.

3. Though, as Socrates notes, philosophy begins with opinions. Nonetheless, philosophy is the attempt to replace opinions with knowledge, to ascend from the cave to the truth. Similarly, Aristotle notes that virtue is related to human nature as act is related to potency. The act cannot be known by starting from potency, rather, potency becomes known by looking back to it from the act.

4. For Aristotle, ethics and politics are a special type of knowledge, *phronesis*, the end of which is not a product that exists outside of human life or a contemplative theory. Rather, these practical sciences have as their end the human activity of leading a good life. As these pursuits involve choice, disagreement, and change, Aristotle notes that the practical sciences are not as precise as theoretical knowledge.

5. By contrast, the Epicureans identified the good with pleasure, although they did not have a base account of pleasure.

6. "And the Lord said, 'Behold, they are one people, and they have all one language; and this is only the beginning of what they will do; and nothing that they propose to do will now be impossible for them" (Gen. 11:1–9).

7. Socrates hid his head when discussing matters of eugenics, perhaps in recognition of how shameful such policies would be in practice, no matter how ideal they are "in speech."

8. For Socrates, it would be more accurate to speak of the self as an "imprisoned" rather than an "embodied" soul. Mary Midgley (1978) sees in Plato the roots of the modern dismissive attitude toward human "brute" or "animal" nature.

9. The Psalm goes on to read, "nevertheless, you will die like men."

10. Genesis states that humans were made in the "image and likeness" of God. In the Fall, humans lost the likeness of God, as they were no longer perfect and perfectly in harmony with their world.

11. For example, the first word in the Rule of St. Benedict is, "Listen."

12. Martin Heidegger (1977) makes the same point that modern physics prepared the way for the essence of technology, which is a "challenging" revealing of nature as mere "standing reserve."

13. As Hobbes was to later put the matter, we can only know those things that we create. Wisdom is the same as free construction. But the control of nature does not require the understanding of nature, meaning there are no limits to the human conquest of nature.

14. This promise was celebrated by Auguste Comte, whose "positivism" promised at last (after the failures of theology and metaphysics) to rationalize politics.

15. This is so, because the living organism testifies to the interrelatedness of spirit and matter. The dualism was therefore resolved into alternate monisms, each of which sought to reduce the other pole under its own principles.

16. Kant's autonomy culminates in Rawlsian liberalism, where individuals determine what is good for them. To be self-governing is to be governed by one's own desires and conceptions of the good, leaving no place for others to shape these motivations.

17. Thus we see the origins of not only the liberal political rights-based doctrine, but also the unfettered pursuit of private preferences that defines capitalism. The latter aspect of the modern condition is an equal consequence of shifting from the notion of the self as a functional part of the natural order to the notion of the autonomous self.

18. The individual became the origin of the moral world, "since man — as distinguished from man's end — had become that center or origin" (Strauss 1953, 248).

19. Though the groundwork for this position was laid in the seventeenth century, it did not blossom until the mid-twentieth century arrival of Keynesian economics, which accepted existing consumer preferences and regulated the economy

by manipulating aggregate demand. As President John F. Kennedy noted in a 1962 commencement address at Yale, "What is at stake in our economic decisions today is not some grand warfare of rival ideologies which will sweep the country with passion but the practical management of a modern economy."

20. Examples of communities for Engelhardt include Orthodox Jews, Eastern Orthodox Christians, Roman Catholics, and Maoist communists.

21. This is so because "in secular philosophical reasoning, ultimate questions cannot be answered" (Englehart 1996, 11). Secularization (like historicism) is the temporalization of the eternal, or the understanding that the eternal is no longer eternal.

THREE   **In Defense of Rich Public Bioethics I: Self and Society**

1. There is an ontological distinction between the council's analysis and this point about equity and autonomy. The council primarily focuses on human nature as defined by intrinsic qualities and capacities. This point about assemblages casts humans as socially defined by extrinsic circumstances. Both ways of looking provide important insights. Unfortunately, many proponents of the social-constructivist approach dismiss human nature as mere myth.

2. Most important human relations are clearly not done justice through the language of "contracts." A family, for example, is a rich composite of mutual care, not a compendium of transactions to be tallied in terms of costs and benefits to the parties involved.

3. Aristotle notes that in order to perform right actions, "the agent must be in a certain condition when he does them; in the first place he must have knowledge, secondly he must choose the acts, and choose them for their own sakes, and thirdly his action must proceed from a firm and unchangeable character" (*Nicomachean Ethics*, 1104a).

4. The creation of ethics advisory bodies requires tax dollars, so in this minimal sense it is a coercive act to use taxpayer money to support a kind of inquiry that not everyone likes. But this degree of coercion is insignificant when compared with other controversial uses of taxpayer dollars, including those that go to the conduct of war.

5. Mary Anderlik Majunder (2005) interpreted the council as striking both anti-democratic and democratic poses—as being exclusionary in advancing a dogmatic vision in some reports, while being tolerant in fostering a more reasonable democratic discourse in others.

6. Stephen Toulmin (2001) similarly defends a broader conception of reason; so do those who defend "wide reflective equilibrium" (e.g., Van Der Burg and van Willigenburg 1998).

7. As just one example, the Executive Summary reads: "Beyond the issue of the safety of the procedure, however, NBAC found that concerns relating to the

potential psychological harms to children and effects on the moral, religious, and cultural values of society merited further reflection and deliberation" (NBAC 1997, iii).

8. The council also noted that it was responding to a similar call in the other major federal report on cloning, the National Academies of Science Committee on Science, Engineering, and Public Policy (NAS) *Scientific and Medical Aspects of Human Reproductive Cloning* (NAS 2002). That report considers only the scientific and medical aspects of cloning.

9. The majority recommended a ban on cloning-to-produce-children and a four-year moratorium on cloning-for-biomedical-research, whereas the minority recommended a ban on the former and regulation for the latter. The majority consisted of Rebecca Dresser, Francis Fukuyama, Robert George, Mary Ann Glendon, Alfonso Gómez-Lobo, William Hurlbut, Leon Kass, Charles Krauthammer, Paul McHugh, and Gilbert Meilaender. The minority consisted of Elizabeth Blackburn, Daniel Foster, Michael Gazzaniga, William May, Janet Rowley, Michael Sandel, and James Wilson.

10. This insight has been more generally formulated in arguments that "clear and present danger" is not the only kind of harm individuals or society can suffer.

11. *Taking Care* notes, "The defining characteristic of our time seems to be that we are both younger longer and older longer" (Kass Council 2005b, 6).

12. The report notes, "The need to face aging and death—our own and that of our loved ones—with clear minds, caring hearts, and human solidarity reminds us that virtue has not become obsolete in our high-tech world" (23–24).

13. This mirrors a classical Aristotelian critique of the limits of Kantian principles. For more on the practical reasoning involved in ethical decisions see Julia Annas (2001).

14. Chapter 4 especially unbrackets substantive questions, presenting detailed arguments for and against difficult decisions in different circumstances, including foregoing treatment.

FOUR   **In Defense of Rich Public Bioethics II: Mind and Body**

This chapter draws from earlier work in Adam Briggle, "The U.S. President's Council on Bioethics: Modeling a Thicker Knowledge Politics," *Innovation: The European Journal of Social Science Research* 22, no. 1 (March 2009): 35–51.

1. See Deryck Beyleveld and Roger Brownsword (2001) for a related discussion of "dignity as empowerment" and "dignity as constraint."

2. In one sense, my Aristotelian argument in this chapter falls under the same umbrella as Kantianism if "perfectionism" is defined broadly as a moral theory that holds that certain properties constitute human nature and that the good life develops those properties to a high degree (see Hurka 1993). The difference,

of course, lies in which properties are designated as ethically relevant to human flourishing. I claim that a wider set of properties, including those tied to human biological nature, is ethically important.

3. I do not maintain that all Kantians suffer under my objections. In fact, Christine Korsgaard (1996) develops a blended Kantian-Aristotelian theory of reflective endorsement that is very similar to my position.

4. See Kant's doctrine of "the two standpoints" in *Fundamental Principles of the Metaphysics of Morals* (1785).

5. As for becoming cyborgs via biotechnological tinkering, human nature, like a rainforest ecosystem, is simply too complex to survive radical transformation (Arnhart 1998; Arnhart 2003). If we were wholly self-making creatures, there would not be a problem here.

6. Francis Fukuyama (2002) makes the same argument, by showing that modern liberal theorists from Kant to Rawls "end up reinserting various assumptions about human nature into their theories" (120).

7. As one historian of ethics put Hume's position, "It is a neutral universe and only our response to it makes it otherwise. If our approval is what makes some motives good, others bad, then we are not subject to error as we would be if we had to know an objective Order in God's mind, or an objective degree of perfection" (Schneewind 1998, 524).

8. For Hume, "reason is, and ought only to be, the slave of the passions, and can never pretend to any office, other than to serve and obey them" (*Treatise of Human Nature* 1740, II, 3, iii). Of course, Hume had a more nuanced view, but I am using him to articulate the widespread assumptions that are necessary for the naturalistic fallacy.

9. Arnhart similarly argues that the fact/value dichotomy can be bridged by identifying the good as the desirable: but not all desires are good, only those that lead to a flourishing life. Midgley adds the complementary point that something is bad if it ruins the whole shape of a life. Aggression, for example, is bound up with central structure of feelings and is thus involved with the development of many valuable parts of life. To attempt to remove such central factors would be disastrous, because the whole complex would collapse. This, of course, is not the same as arguing that all instances of aggression are good.

10. This would be what John Finnis (1980) called the "illicit inference from facts to norms."

11. Midgley makes the same point that we cannot get rid of the value judgment in talking about adaptations—they tell us that "this is the good which x does." To replace talk of adaptations (a seal is adapted to cut through water) with neutral-looking formulas such as (a seal has no trouble cutting through water) is to lose the explanatory point (Midgley 1978, 74).

12. It is worth noting that even Michel Foucault, whose work inspires so many postmodern deniers of the natural body, wrote of the "inscription" of cul-

tural practices *on a natural body,* which he described in terms of force, materiality, energy, sensation, and pleasure.

13. Bostrom seems to believe that the only possible normative appeal to nature is of the kind lampooned by J. S. Mill, namely, assertions that whatever is natural is good. He points out that malaria and murder are obviously both natural and bad. In so doing, he somehow thinks he has successfully dismissed the natural law tradition, at least as Kass (e.g., 1996) interprets it, but he has only defeated his own straw man.

14. The quotations refer to Norton's paraphrasing from Leo Strauss (1953).

15. This insight is developed in Jonas's ontological investigation of life and the living organism (1966). Far from being the achievement of a disembodied will, identity as a self is made possible only through the metabolic workings of the body. The metabolic process signals not just new patterns of material exchange. It is also already and always the essence of identity and interiority that comprise consciousness or selfhood.

16. A similar argument can be found in Bill McKibben (2003).

17. Though such a radical dystopia may not emerge, intimations already exist of the outcomes that worried Huxley—for example, the growing medicalization of society (see Elliott 1999).

18. Bostrom (2005) provides just one example of an unreflective and simplistic proposal to eradicate those "thoroughly unrespectable and unacceptable" aspects of our "species-specific nature," as if this ontological surgery could occur without influencing more "respectable and acceptable" aspects of human nature.

19. This is one way to summarize the primary justification for a rich public bioethics. The council put it a slightly different way in their report *Being Human*: "We are quick to notice dangers to life, threats to freedom, and risks of discrimination or exploitation. But we are slow to think about the need to uphold human dignity and the many ways of doing and feeling and being in the world that make human life rich, deep, and fulfilling. Indeed, it sometimes seems as though our views of the meaning of our humanity have been so transformed by the technological approach to the world that we may be in danger of forgetting what we have to lose, humanly speaking. To enlarge our vision and deepen our understanding, we need to focus not only on the astonishing new technologies but also on those (in truth, equally astonishing) aspects of 'being human'" (Kass Council 2003b, xx).

F I V E **The Kass Council as Institution and Lightning Rod**

1. Throughout this section, citations are often listed after member and staff names with the purpose of pointing the reader to sources that demonstrate the basic viewpoints of members and staff.

2. This panel authored *Assessing Biomedical Technologies,* one of the first overviews of the moral and social questions posed by biomedical science.

3. The role that "lay" members could play on ethics committees is unclear. Some maintain they are an important way to increase the democratic representativeness of ethics commissions, while others argue they do little more than serve a symbolic function in an attempt to create the appearance of inclusiveness (see Brown 2006; Brown 2008).

4. In this work, Glendon argues that modern American culture lacks the political lexicon and moral vocabulary for expressing normative concepts central to public life.

5. In the April 25, 2002, session Gazzaniga defended the principle of scientific self-policing: ". . . let the scientists roll. They'll figure it out." Krauthammer took issue with this, raising the "slippery slope argument" as a justification for greater control. Wilson took issue with that argument, precipitating some of the most heated debate.

6. The council operated under a variety of federal statutes and regulations, most notably the Federal Advisory Committee Act, or FACA (1972), the Ethics in Government Act (1978), and the Freedom of Information Act (1966). In general, these statutes are designed to ensure accountability and transparency. FACA is particularly important, because it articulates certain principles for advisory committees and sets guidelines for their creation and management. The General Services Administration (GSA) is responsible for implementing FACA rules. For more on this, see chapter 6.

7. This "distortion" of ethical reflection needs to be carefully defined and distinguished from the inevitable and even beneficial political elements of bioethics commissions. I undertake this analysis in the next chapter, drawing from norms of independence, balance, and transparency.

8. Fletcher and Miller (writing before NBAC and the Kass Council) maintained that political co-optation had not occurred in public bioethics, outside of the crippling effects of the abortion controversy on BEAC.

9. This is the third in a series of NAS reports to the U.S. presidents, each issued in an election year.

10. In a twist on Kass's fears of Huxley's dystopia, these bioethicists suggest that an Orwellian dystopia may result from the mentality of Kass and Bush. Caplan (2004) also took issue with the council's overly pessimistic portrayal of biomedical progress, arguing that the council's attitude could be a discouragement to finding urgently needed cures.

11. At the first meeting (January 17, 2002), George applauded "the President's willingness to appoint to the Council not only people who agree with his fundamental moral outlook on the questions before us, but also some who don't and some who deviate very, very sharply indeed from the President's own perspective."

12. There was a gradation of viewpoints within both the majority and minority "coalitions." As is evidenced in the report and in the transcripts, three members (Fukuyama, McHugh, and Dresser) wanted a moratorium only until adequate regulations were drawn up. Thus the actual vote of the council could be read as 10-7 in favor of cloning-for-biomedical-research, rather than the other way around (see Saletan 2002).

13. One remark by Kass in this regard comes from the April 25, 2002, session on cloning: "We don't want to simply decide on the basis of the wisdom of the vote of the majority to silence any arguments sincerely held and properly defended. It might very well be that an argument made and held by one person is the best argument and we would deprive our readers of the benefit of having to weigh that."

14. See Brock (1987) for an overview of the tensions inherent in these terms tailored to federal bioethics commissions.

15. Indeed at their final meeting, Fukuyama expressed disappointment in the council's failure to make a larger impact on biomedical science and technology regulations. But Saletan (2005) argued that the council was finally coming around to addressing urgent, practical issues by the end of Kass's tenure as chair.

S I X   **The Politicization of Ethics Advice**

This chapter draws from earlier work in Adam Briggle, "The Kass Council and the Politicization of Ethics Advice," *Social Studies of Science*, vol. 39, no. 2 (April 2009): 309–26.

1. I use the term "science" here to denote empirical processes striving for systematic knowledge of nature.

2. The opposite is also true, namely, that an advisory body may in fact be doing a poor job of upholding the relevant norms, but still achieve legitimacy because it successfully dupes its audiences into believing that it is upholding the norms. This seems a less likely scenario, however, and does not apply to the council.

3. Others point out epistemological analogues between scientific and ethical expertise that would make this parallel even stronger (Singer 1972; Annas 2002).

4. This is especially true given the council's mandated freedom from consensus and tendency to tackle questions of the moral "good" more so than the "right." On these matters, as Kass said in his opening remarks (Jan. 17, 2002), "reasonable and morally serious people can differ."

5. In a related formulation, David Cash and others defined legitimacy as the conduct of advice and public discussion that is perceived to be "respectful of stakeholders' divergent values and beliefs, unbiased in its conduct, and fair in its treatment of opposing views and interests" (2003, 8086).

6. At this point my thought experiment deviates from Pielke. He considers stealth issue advocacy as occurring when a scientist pretends to be a "pure scientist" but is in fact an issue advocate. I could portray criticisms of the Kass Council ,as arising from expectations that it was supposed to be a "pure ethics panel" or "ethics arbiter." But the above formulation works just as well and is simpler.

7. Other members were also released but without much controversy, though it is unclear if it was William May's choice to step down (see Kohn and Bell 2004).

8. Stephen Hall, a reporter for *Science,* suggested that this controversy tainted what was otherwise arguably "the most wide-ranging, in-depth and thoughtful public discussion of the cloning issue in the United States" (Hall 2002, 322). He continued: "In the end, the council's last-minute majority might have spared the president considerable embarrassment, but at a price: the possible loss of long-term credibility" (324).

9. Upon seeing the majority position change from what appeared to be a pro-cloning view to the recommendation of a moratorium, Rowley said she was "really caught by surprise," and Gazzaniga advocated for further clarification of the moratorium position than was ultimately provided. Kass argued that there was nothing manufactured about the majority.

SEVEN   **The Kass Council as Humanities Policy**

1. The ratio of NSF to NEH funding went from 5:1 in 1979 to 33:1 in 1997 (Frodeman, Pielke, and Mitcham 2003).

2. This is why "impact" is not universally recognized as the only criterion of success for bioethics committees. Indeed, one survey of bioethics committees around the world noted that their most important contributions are often the intangible efforts to "enhance the debate between science, the world of politics and the public" (Fuchs 2005, 92). The same report observed that "here are institutions such as the Danish Council that are internationally regarded as successful although they have not manifestly influenced actual political decisions" (91).

3. In an implicit plea for humanities policy, Sarewitz concludes that "the values bases of disputes . . . must be fully articulated and adjudicated . . . before science can play an effective role in resolving" science policy disputes (2004, 385).

4. The so-called "third wave" of science studies is a counterweight to this relativist trend. Its proponents seek to save politics from an illusory utopian rationalism while nonetheless protecting a moderate pragmatic rationalism grounded in the epistemic value of expert knowledge.

5. Prior to this, the 1880 Allison Commission was an important development in the governance of U.S. publicly funded science. Some of the first modern "science policy" works are *The Prince* (1513) and the *New Atlantis* (1624), which tells a fable that foreshadows the post–World War II notion that science and society must be kept separate.

6. Science policy research refers to the literature generated by those who study science policy practices such as federal budgets for research and development.

7. Most notably, in *The New Politics of Science* (1984) David Dickson argued against the narrowing of science policy. In explicitly normative and populist terms, Dickson argued that national science policy had removed decision-making power from the public and placed it in the hands of corporate, military, and political elites.

8. For example, Kuehn and Porter claim that science "must provide the social link between ends and means" (1981, 19). They defined the goals of science policy as "the application of technology to satisfy human needs" (12). They also noted health as another rationale for public investment in science, but even this goal is often subsumed under the rubric of economics. This is especially apparent in the growing commercialization of pharmacology and other biologics.

9. Stokes's concern is just with the relationship between science (understanding) and use (technology). He does not consider the worthiness of different uses or the ethical and societal implications of the resulting technologies. Stokes acknowledges the occasional requirement for "the analysis of complex moral and ethical issues," but he dismisses these cases as exceptions to the rule (1997, 115). Thus, he marginalizes or ignores judgments of social value of scientific knowledge and technological applications.

10. Guston's focus is on the productivity and integrity of science. This latter category is about the proper means for acquiring knowledge, not the proper knowledge to acquire.

11. This is evident, for example, in the 1980 Bayh-Dole Act, which promoted the licensing of patents from publicly funded research by allowing universities, the Office of Technology Transfer at the National Institutes of Health, the Advanced Technology Program at the National Institute of Standards and Technology, University-Industry Research Centers, and the National Bureau of Standards Experimental Technology Incentives Program to retain title to their inventions.

12. Though some argue that these connections are tenuous and poorly understood at best, U.S. science policies tend to be driven by such claims of how growing investments in science will solve national crises of all sorts, including economic competitiveness (see Lucena 2005).

13. One could see this foreshadowed by Vannevar Bush: "It would be folly to set up a program under which research in the natural sciences and medicine was expanded at the cost of the social sciences, humanities, and other studies so essential to national well-being" (1945, 18). Similarly, Bush later compiled some of his essays in a volume entitled *Science Is Not Enough* (1967).

14. The ideal of the social sciences is descriptive knowledge in the form of lawlike generalizations with strong predictive power (see MacIntyre 1984).

15. Fuller (2000) draws a similar distinction between "liberal science policy," which involves attempts to satisfy individual preferences without positing a civic

ideal, and a "republican science policy," which is akin to my concept of rich science policy. See also Frodeman and Mitcham (2000).

16. This is of course only a descriptive point and not a normative claim about cultural relativism.

17. This quotation from *Democracy in America* can be found in the edition by Bruce Frohnen, translator Henry Reeve 2003.

18. Taylor (1989) similarly likens the philosopher, critic, or scientist to the mechanic in the pit, while the artist is the race-car driver. Only art can *realize* the sources of "personal resonance" and make contact with truth and meaning.

Conclusion

1. Stephen Toulmin (1982) argued that medical ethics and other practical or applied ethics "saved the life of ethics." Practical ethics is a much needed response to the inadequacies of metaethics and the formalization of decision theoretic procedures. Especially over the last third of the twentieth century, these approaches offered no assistance to societies facing the substantive issues presented by the creation and use of technology.

2. Kitcher argues that only once "we require an estimate of the chances the desired outcomes will be delivered [is it] appropriate to turn at this point to groups of experts" (2001, 119)

3. It could also be seen as an expression of the contemporary revival of republicanism. For example, Sandel (1996) argues that the shortcomings of liberalism require a "political economy of citizenship." This means not just sharing in self-rule, but "deliberating with fellow citizens about the common good and helping to shape the destiny of the political community" (58). Sharing in self-rule "requires that citizens possess, or come to acquire, certain civic virtues. But this means that republican politics cannot be neutral toward the values and ends its citizens espouse. The republican conception of freedom, unlike the liberal conception, requires a formative politics, a politics that cultivates in citizens the qualities of character that self-government requires" (58).

4. Indeed, to treat truth as a direct, personal vision of being is to make it so subjective as to have no way of distinguishing philosophers (reason) from lunatics or the authority of the ancestors.

5. This accusation continued to be leveled at the Pellegrino Council. For example, as an invited guest to a Pellegrino Council meeting (March 7, 2008), Stephen Pinker criticized *Human Dignity and Bioethics* for being insufficiently representative of relevant viewpoints, including those from "mainstream" bioethics and secular traditions. Pinker was certainly right on this point, particularly regarding the absence of an essay from Ruth Macklin or someone defending a view similar to hers.

WORKS CITED

Abram, David. 1996. *The Spell of the Sensuous: Perception and Language in a More-than-Human-World.* New York: Pantheon.

Ackerman, Bruce. 1980. *Social Justice in the Liberal State.* New Haven, CT: Yale University Press.

Agar, Nicholas. 2004. *Liberal Eugenics: In Defence of Human Enhancement.* Malden, MA: Blackwell.

Ahvenharju, Sanna, et al. 2006. *Comparative Analysis of Opinions Produced by National Ethics Councils.* Helsinki, Finland: Gaia Group Ltd.

Ainslie, Donald C. 2004. "Principlism." In *Encyclopedia of Bioethics,* 3rd ed., edited by Stephen Post, 2099–2104. New York: Macmillan.

Alexander, Shana. 1962. "They Decide Who Lives, Who Dies." *Life,* November 9.

American Society for Cell Biology. 2004. "Cell Biologists Oppose Removal of Top Scientist." (March 2). http://www.ascb.org/files%5Cpre-2006_press_releases.pdf.

Anderson, Maria. 2004. "Bush Dismisses Council Members." *Scientist* 5, no. 1 (March 3): 303–4.

Annas, George. 1993. *Standard of Care: The Law of American Bioethics.* New York: Oxford University Press.

Annas, George, and Sherman Elias. 2004. "Politics, Morals, and Embryos." *Nature* 431: 19–20.

Annas, Julia. 2002. "Moral Knowledge as Practical Knowledge." *Social Philosophy and Policy* 18, no. 2: 236–56.

Anscombe, G. E. M. 1958. "Modern Moral Philosophy." *Philosophy* 33, no. 124: 1–19.

Appiah, Kwame Anthony. 2005. *The Ethics of Identity.* Princeton, NJ: Princeton University Press.

Arendt, Hannah. 1958. *The Human Condition.* Chicago: University of Chicago Press.

Aristotle. 1992. *Eudemian Ethics.* Edited by Michael Woods. Oxford: Oxford University Press.

Arnhart, Larry. 1998. *Darwinian Natural Right: The Biological Ethics of Human Nature.* Albany, NY: State University of New York Press.

———. 2003. "Human Nature Is Here to Stay." *New Atlantis,* no. 2 (Summer): 65–78.

————. 2005. "President's Council on Bioethics." In *Encyclopedia of Science, Technology, and Ethics,* edited by Carl Mitcham, 1482–86. New York: Macmillan.

Arrow, Kenneth. 1951. *Social Choice and Individual Values.* New York: Wiley.

Asch, Adrienne. 2005. "Big Tent Bioethics: Toward an Inclusive and Reasonable Bioethics." *Hastings Center Report* 35, no. 6: 11–12.

Bacon, Francis. 1999. *Selected Philosophical Works.* Edited by Rose-Mary Sargent. Indianapolis, IN: Hackett.

Barry, Brian. 1965. *Political Argument.* London: Routledge and Kegan Paul.

Beauchamp, Tom, and James Childress. 1979. *Principles of Biomedical Ethics.* 1st ed. New York: Oxford University Press.

Beauchamp, Tom, and LeRoy Walters. 2003. *Contemporary Issues in Bioethics.* 6th ed. Belmont, CA: Wadsworth-Thompson Learning.

Beecher, Henry. 1966. "Ethics and Clinical Research." *New England Journal of Medicine* 274: 1354–60.

Berkowitz, Peter. 1999. *Virtue and the Making of Modern Liberalism.* Princeton, NJ: Princeton University Press.

————. 2002. "Pathos of the Kass Report." *Policy Review,* October/November, 71–79.

————. 2003. *Never a Matter of Indifference: Sustaining Virtue in a Free Republic.* Stanford, CA: Hoover Institution.

Berlin, Isaiah. 1998. *The Crooked Timber of Humanity.* Edited by Henry Hardy. Princeton, NJ: Princeton University Press.

Beyleveld, Deryck, and Roger Brownsword. 2001. *Human Dignity in Bioethics and Biolaw.* Oxford: Oxford University Press.

Bimber, Bruce. 1996. *The Politics of Expertise in Congress: The Rise and Fall of the Office of Technology Assessment.* Albany, NY: State University of New York Press.

Blackburn, Elizabeth. 2004a. "Bioethics and the Political Distortion of Biomedical Science." *New England Journal of Medicine* 350, no. 14: 1379–80.

————. 2004b. "A 'Full Range' of Bioethical Views Just Got Narrower." *Washington Post,* March 7.

————. 2005. "Thoughts of a Former Council Member." *Perspectives in Biology and Medicine* 48, no. 2: 172–80.

Blackburn, Elizabeth, and Janet Rowley. 2004. "Reason as Our Guide." Public Library of Science *Biology* 2, no. 4: 420–22.

Blackford, Russell. 2005. "The Supposed Sin of Defying Nature." Institute for Ethics and Emerging Technologies, January 19 and 26. http://www.ieet.org/.

Blank, Robert. 1994. "A National Forum for Bioethics: Attractive But Unworkable or Workable But Unattractive." *Politics and the Life Sciences* 13: 77–78.

Borgmann, Albert. 1984. *Technology and the Character of Contemporary Life.* Chicago: University of Chicago Press.

———. 2006. "Mediating Between Science and Technology." In *Postphenomenology: A Critical Companion to Ihde*, edited by Evan Selinger, 247–55. Albany, NY: State University of New York Press.

Bostrom, Nick. 2004. "Transhumanism: The World's Most Dangerous Idea?" *Foreign Affairs* (September/October).

———. 2005. "In Defense of Posthuman Dignity." *Bioethics* 19, no. 3: 202–14.

Bozeman, Barry, and Daniel Sarewitz. 2005. "Public-Value Failure: When Efficient Markets May Not Do." *Public Administration Review* 62, no. 2: 134–51.

Breck, John, and Lyn Breck. 2005. *Stages on Life's Way: Orthodox Thinking on Bioethics*. Crestwood, NY: St. Vladimir's Seminary Press.

Briggle, Adam. 2009a. "The U.S. President's Council on Bioethics: Modeling a Thicker Knowledge Politics." *Innovation: The European Journal of Social Science Research* 22, no. 1, March: 35–51.

———. 2009b. "The Kass Council and the Politicization of Ethics Advice." *Social Studies of Science* 39, no. 2, April: 309–26.

Briggle, Adam, Robert Frodeman, and J. Britt Holbrook. 2006. "Introducing a Policy Turn in *Environmental Philosophy*." *Environmental Philosophy* 3, no. 1: 70–77.

Briggle, Adam, and Carl Mitcham. 2009. "The Embedded and the Networked: Conceptualizing Technology-Society Experience." *Technology in Society* 31: 374–83.

Brink, David. 1989. *Moral Realism and the Foundations of Ethics*. New York: Cambridge University Press.

Brock, Dan. 1987. "Truth or Consequences: The Role of Philosophers in Policy-Making." *Ethics* 97, no. 4: 786–91.

———. 2004. "Public Policy and Bioethics." In *Encyclopedia of Bioethics*, 3rd ed., edited by Stephen Post, 2234–42. New York: Macmillan.

Brooks, Harvey. 1996. "The Evolution of U.S. Science Policy." In *Technology, R&D, and the Economy*, edited by Bruce Smith and Claude Barfield, 15–48. Washington, DC: Brookings Institution.

Brown, Mark. 2006. "Ethics, Politics, and the Public: Shaping the Research Agenda." In *Shaping Science & Technology Policy: The Next Generation of Research*, edited by David Guston and Daniel Satewitz, 10–32. Madison, WI: University of Wisconsin Press.

———. 2008. "Three Ways to Politicize Bioethics." *American Journal of Bioethics*.

Burt, Robert. 2005. "The End of Autonomy," *Hastings Center Report* 35, no. 6: S9–S13.

Bush, Vannevar. 1945. *Science—The Endless Frontier: A Report to the President on a Program for Postwar Scientific Research*. Washington, DC: National Science Foundation.

———. 1967. *Science is Not Enough*. New York: Morrow.

Callahan, Daniel. 1973. "Bioethics as a Discipline." *Hastings Center Studies* 1: 66–73.

————. 1998. *False Hopes: Why America's Quest for Perfect Health Is a Recipe for Failure*. New York: Simon and Schuster.

————. 2003. "Individual Good and Common Good: A Communitarian Approach to Bioethics." *Perspectives in Biology and Medicine* 46, no. 4: 496–507.

————. 2004. "Bioethics." In *Encyclopedia of Bioethics*, 3rd ed., edited by Stephen Post, 278–87. New York: Macmillan.

Cameron, Nigel. 2002. "Defending Dignity: An Interview with Leon Kass." *American Enterprise* 13, no. 7: 44–46.

Caplan, Arthur. 2002. "A Council of Clones." *Diabetes Daily News*, January 18.

Carmen, Ira. 1994. "Bioethics, Public Policy, and Political Science." *Politics and the Life Sciences* 13: 79–81.

Carson, Benjamin. 1992. *Think Big: Unleashing Your Potential for Excellence*. Grand Rapids, MI: Zondervan.

Carson, Rachel. 1962. *Silent Spring*. Boston: Houghton Mifflin.

Cash, David, et al. 2003. "Knowledge Systems for Sustainable Development." *Proceedings of the National Academy of Sciences* 100, no. 14: 8086–91.

Chambers, Tod. 1999. *The Fiction of Bioethics: Cases as Literary Texts*. New York: Routledge.

Charo, R. Alta. 2004. "Passing on the Right: Conservative Bioethics Is Closer Than It Appears." *Journal of Law, Medicine, and Ethics* 32: 307–14.

————. 2007. "The Endarkenment." In *The Ethics of Bioethics: Mapping the Moral Landscape*, edited by Lisa Eckenwiler and Felicia Cohn, 95–107. Baltimore, MD: Johns Hopkins University Press.

Charon, Rita, and Martha Montello. 2005. *Stories Matter: The Role of Narrative in Medical Ethics*. New York: Routledge.

Childress, James. 1970. "Who Shall Live When Not All Can Live?" *Soundings* 53: 339–55.

Clement, Grace. 1996. *Care, Autonomy, and Justice: Feminism and the Ethic of Care*. Boulder, CO: Westview Press.

Clouser, K. Danner, and Bernard Gert. 1990. "A Critique of Principlism." *Journal of Medicine and Philosophy* 152: 219–36.

Cohen, Cynthia. 1994. "Searching for a Variety of Bioethics Forums." *Politics and the Life Sciences* 13: 82–84.

————. 2005a. "The President's Council on Bioethics and Approaches to Public Deliberation Taken by National Bioethics Commissions." *Kennedy Institute of Ethics Journal* 15, no. 3: 219–20.

————. 2005b. "Promises and Perils of Public Deliberation: Contrasting Two National Bioethics Commissions on Embryonic Stem Cell Research." *Kennedy Institute of Ethics Journal* 15, no. 3: 269–88.

Cohen, Eric. 2004. "Science, Democracy, and Stem Cells." *Philosophy Today* 48, no. 5: 23–29.

————. 2006. "Conservative Bioethics and the Search for Wisdom," *Hastings Center Report* 36, no. 1: 44–56.

Collins, H. M., and Robert Evans. 2006. "The Third Wave of Science Studies: Studies of Expertise and Experience." In *The Philosophy of Expertise*, edited by Evan Selinger and Robert Crease, 39–110. New York: Columbia University Press.

Cook, Michael. 2004. "Ethics as Our Guide." Public Library of Science *Biology* 2, no. 6: 737.

Dahl, Robert. 1998. *On Democracy*. New Haven, CT: Yale University Press.

Davis, R. B. 1995. "The Principlism Debate: A Critical Overview." *Journal of Medicine and Philosophy* 20, no. 1: 85–105.

Deephouse, David L., and Suzanne M. Carter. 2005. "An Examination of Differences between Organizational Legitimacy and Organizational Reputation." *Journal of Management Studies* 42, no. 2: 329–60.

Descartes, René. [1637] 1998. *Discourse on Method*. Translated by Donald A. Cress. Indianapolis, IN: Hackett.

de Tocqueville, Alexis. [1835] 2003. *Democracy in America*. Edited by Bruce Frohnen. Translated by Henry Reeve. Washington, DC: Regnery Gateway.

Diamond, Cora. 1991. *The Realistic Spirit: Wittgenstein, Philosophy, and the Mind*. Cambridge, MA: Bradford Books.

———. 1996. "Wittgenstein, Mathematics, and Ethics: Resisting the Attractions of Realism." In *Cambridge Companion to Wittgenstein*, edited by Hans D. Sluga and David G. Stern, 226–60. Cambridge: Cambridge University Press.

———. 2006. "The Difficulty of Reality and the Difficulty of Philosophy." In *Reading Cavell*, edited by Alice Crary and Sanford Shieh, 98–118. London: Routledge.

Dickson, David. 1984. *The New Politics of Science*. New York: Pantheon.

Dresser, Rebecca. 2003. "Precommitment: A Misguided Strategy for Securing Death with Dignity." Symposium on Precommitment Theory, Bioethics, and Constitutional Law, *Texas Law Review* 81: 1823–47.

———. 2005. Telephone interview by Adam Briggle. December 9.

Dupree, A. Hunter. 1957. *Science in the Federal Government: A History of Policies and Activities to 1940*. Cambridge, MA: Belknap Press.

Dworkin, Ronald. 1989. "The Concept of Autonomy." In *The Inner Citadel*, edited by John Christman, 54–62. New York: Oxford University Press.

Dzur, Albert, and Daniel Levin. 2004. "The 'Nation's Conscience': Assessing Bioethics Commissions as Public Forums." *The Kennedy Institute of Ethics Journal* 14, no. 4: 333–60.

———. 2007. "The Primacy of the Public: In Support of Bioethics Commissions as Deliberative Forums." *Kennedy Institute of Ethics Journal* 17, no. 2: 133–42.

Easterbrook, Gregg. 2003. *The Progress Paradox: How Life Gets Better While People Feel Worse*. New York: Random House.

Eiseman, Elisa. 2003. *The National Bioethics Advisory Commission: Contributing to Public Policy*. Arlington, VA: RAND.

Ellen, Ruth, Elizabeth Meyer Bobby, and Harvey Fineberg, eds. 1995. *Society's Choices: Social and Ethical Decision Making in Biomedicine*. A Report by the Institute of Medicine, Committee on the Social and Ethical Impacts of Developments in Biomedicine. Washington, DC: National Academies Press.

Elliott, Carl. 1999. *A Philosophical Disease: Bioethics, Culture, and Identity*. New York: Routledge.

———. 2003. *Better than Well: American Medicine Meets the American Dream*. New York: W.W. Norton.

———. 2004. "Beyond Politics." *MSN Slate Magazine*, March 9. http://www .slate.com/.

———. 2008. "Guinea-pigging." *New Yorker* 83, no. 42 (January 7): 36–41.

Engelhardt, Tristram, Jr. 1996. *The Foundations of Bioethics*. 2nd ed. New York: Oxford University Press.

Evans, John. 2002. *Playing God? Human Genetic Engineering and the Rationalization of Public Bioethical Debate*. Chicago: University of Chicago Press.

———. 2006. "Between Technocracy and Democratic Legitimation: A Proposed Compromise Position for Common Morality Public Bioethics." *Journal of Medicine and Philosophy* 31: 213–34.

Ezrahi, Yaron. 1990. *The Descent of Icarus: Science and the Transformation of Contemporary Democracy*. London: Harvard University Press.

Fagerlin, Angela, and Carl. E. Schneider. 2004. "Enough: The Failure of the Living Will." In *Bioethics: An Introduction to the History, Methods, and Practice*, 2nd ed., edited by Nancy Jecker, Albert Jonsen, and Robert Pearlman, 440–56. Boston: Jones and Bartlett.

Feenberg, Andrew. 1991. *Critical Theory of Technology*. Oxford: Oxford University Press.

Ferguson, Andrew. 2002. "Kass Warfare: The President's Bioethics Council Enters the Cloning Fray." *Weekly Standard* 7, no. 20: 13–15.

Finnis, John. 1980. *Natural Law and Natural Rights*. Oxford: Oxford University Press.

Fish, Stanley. 2008. "Will the Humanities Save Us?" *New York Times*, January 6.

Fleming, Donald. 1969. "On Living in a Biological Revolution." *Atlantic Monthly* 223, no. 2 (February): 64–70.

Fletcher, John. 1994. "On Restoring Public Bioethics." *Politics and the Life Sciences* 13: 84–86.

Fletcher, John, and Franklin Miller. 1996. "The Promise and Perils of Public Bioethics." In *The Ethics of Research Involving Human Subjects: Facing the 21st Century*, edited by Harold Vanderpool, 155–84. Frederick, MD: University Publishing Group.

Flitner, David, Jr. 1986. *The Politics of Presidential Commissions*. Dobbs Ferry, NY: Transnational Publishers.

Fox, Renèe, and Judith Swazey. 2008. *Observing Bioethics*. Oxford: Oxford University Press.

Frankfurt, Harry. 2004. *The Reasons of Love.* Princeton, NJ: Princeton University Press.

Frodeman, Robert. 2003. *Geo-Logic: Breaking Ground Between Philosophy and the Earth Sciences.* Albany, NY: State University of New York Press.

————. 2006. "The Role of Humanities Policy in Public Science." In *Public Science in Liberal Democracy,* edited by Peter Phillips, 111–20. Toronto: University of Toronto Press.

Frodeman, Robert, and Carl Mitcham. 2000. "Beyond the Social Contract Myth: Integrating Science and the Common Good." *Issues in Science and Technology* 16, no. 4: 37–41.

Frodeman, Robert, Carl Mitcham, and Roger Pielke, Jr. 2003. "Humanities Policy— and a Policy for the Humanities." *Issues in Science and Technology* (Fall): 29–32.

Fuchs, Michael. 2005. *National Ethics Councils: Their Backgrounds, Functions, and Modes of Operation Compared.* Berlin: Nationaler Ethikrat.

Fukuyama, Francis. 1992. *The End of History and the Last Man.* New York: Free Press.

————. 2002. *Our Posthuman Future: Consequences of the Biotechnology Revolution.* New York: Farar, Straus and Giroux.

————. 2005. "Human Biomedicine and the Problem of Governance." *Perspectives in Biology and Medicine* 48, no. 2: 195–200.

Fuller, Steve. 2000. *The Governance of Science: Ideology and the Future of the Open Society.* Philadelphia: Open University Press.

Funtowicz, S. O., and J. R. Ravetz. 1993. "Science for the Post-Normal Age." *Futures* 25, no. 7 (Sept.): 735–55.

Galston, William. 2001. "He's Fair and Mainstream." *USA Today,* August 15.

Garreau, Joel. 2006. "A Dose of Genius: 'Smart Pills' Are on the Rise. But Is Taking Them Wise?" *Washington Post* (June 11): D01.

Gazzaniga, Michael. 2004. "Human Being Redux." *Science* 304, no. 5669: 388–89.

————. 2005. *The Ethical Brain.* New York: Dana Press.

————. 2006a. "All Clones Are Not the Same." *New York Times,* February 16.

————. 2006b. Telephone interview by Adam Briggle. July 5.

George, Robert. 1993. *Making Men Moral: Civil Liberties and Public Morality.* Oxford: Clarendon Press.

————. 1999. *In Defense of Natural Law.* Oxford: Clarendon Press.

Gillespie, Nick. 2002. "Anti-Science-Fiction." *MSN Slate Magazine,* January 18. http://www.slate.com/.

Glannon, Walter. 2005. *Biomedical Ethics.* New York: Oxford University Press.

Glendon, Mary Ann. 1991. *Rights Talk: The Impoverishment of Political Discourse.* New York: Free Press.

Gómez-Lobo, Alfonso. 2002. *Morality and the Human Goods: An Introduction to Natural Law Ethics.* Washington, DC: Georgetown University Press.

Gourevitch, Victor, and Michael D. Roth. 1991. *On Tyranny.* New York: Free Press.

Gray, Bradford. 1995. "Bioethics Commissions: What Can We Learn from Past Successes and Failures?" In *Society's Choices: Social and Ethical Decisionmaking in Biomedicine,* A Report by the Institute of Medicine, Committee on the Social and Ethical Impacts of Developments in Biomedicine, edited by Ruth Ellen Bulger, Elizabeth Meyer Bobby, and Harvey V. Fineberg, 261–306. Washington, DC: National Academy Press.

Greenberg, Daniel. 1968. *The Politics of Pure Science.* New York: New American Library. Revised ed. 1999. Chicago: University of Chicago Press. (Page references are to revised edition.)

———. 2001. *Science, Money, and Politics: Political Triumph and Ethical Erosion.* Chicago: University of Chicago Press.

Groopman, Jerome. 2002. "Science Fiction." Comment. *New Yorker* (February 4): 23.

Guston, David. 2000. *Between Politics and Science: Assuring the Integrity and Productivity of Research.* New York: Cambridge University Press.

Guston, David, and Kenneth Keniston. 1994. *The Fragile Contract: University Science and the Federal Government.* Cambridge, MA: MIT Press.

Haldane, J. B. S. 1924. *Daedelus; or, Science and the Future.* New York: E. P. Dutton.

Hall, Stephen. 2002. "President's Bioethics Council Delivers." *Science* 297, no. 5580: 322–24.

Hanna, K. E., R. M. Cook-Deegan, and R. Y. Nishimi. 1993. "Finding a Forum for Bioethics in U.S. Public Policy." *Politics and the Life Sciences* 12: 205–19.

———. 1994. "Bioethics and Public Policy: Still Seeking a Forum." *Politics and the Life Sciences* 13: 102–5.

Haraway, Donna. 1991. *Simians, Cyborgs and Women: The Reinvention of Nature.* New York: Routledge.

Heidegger, Martin. [1954] 1977. "The Question concerning Technology." In *The Question concerning Technology and Other Essays.* Translated by William Lovitt. New York.

Heisenberg, Werner. 1952. *Philosophic Problems of Nuclear Science.* New York: Fawcett.

Hilgartner, Stephen. 2000. *Science on Stage: Expert Advice as Public Drama.* Stanford, CA: Stanford University Press.

Hippocrates. 1959. *Hippocrates.* 2 vols. Translated by W. H. S. Jones. Loeb Classical Library. Cambridge, MA: Harvard University Press.

Hirschman, Albert. 1977. *The Passions and the Interests: Political Arguments for Capitalism before Its Triumph.* Princeton: Princeton University Press.

Hobbes, Thomas. [1651] 1991. *Hobbes: Leviathan.* Edited by Richard Tuck. Cambridge: Cambridge University Press.

Holden, Constance. 2004. "Researchers Blast U.S. Bioethics Panel Shuffle." *Science* 303, no. 5667: 1447.

Holland, Stephen. 2003. *Bioethics: A Philosophical Introduction.* Cambridge: Polity Press.

Holton, Gerald. 1979. "From the Endless Frontier to the Ideology of Limits." In *Limits of Scientific Inquiry,* edited by Gerald Holton and Robert Morison, 227–42. New York: W.W. Norton.

Howard-Jones, Norman. 1982. "Human Experimentation in Historical and Ethical Perspectives." *Social Science Medicine* 1615: 1429–48.

Hudson, Kathy. 2004. "Something Old and Something New." *Hastings Center Report* 34, no. 4: 14–15.

Hume, David. [1740] 2000. *A Treatise of Human Nature.* Edited by David Fate Norman and Mary J. Norton. Oxford, Clarendon Press.

Hurka, Thomas. 1993. *Perfectionism.* New York: Oxford University Press.

Huxley, Aldous. 1932. *Brave New World.* New York: Harper Perennial.

Hyde, Michael. 2001. "Defining 'Human Dignity' in the Debate Over the (Im)-Morality of Physician-Assisted Suicide." *Journal of Medical Humanities* 22, no. 1: 69–82.

Jasanoff, Sheila. 1990. *The Fifth Branch: Science Advisors as Policymakers.* Cambridge, MA: Harvard University Press.

Jecker, Nancy. 1997. "Introduction to the Methods of Bioethics." In *Bioethics: An Introduction to the History, Methods, and Practice,* edited by Nancy Jecker, Albert Jonsen, and Robert Pearlman, 113–25. Boston: Jones and Bartlett.

Johnson, Summer. 2007. "A Rebuttal to Dzur and Levin: Johnson on the Legitimacy and Authority of Bioethics Commissions." *Kennedy Institute of Ethics Journal* 17, no. 2: 143–52.

Jonas, Hans. 1966. *The Phenomenon of Life.* New York: Harper and Row.

———. 1969. "Philosophical Reflections on Experimenting with Human Subjects." *Daedulus* 98, no. 2: 219–47.

Jonsen, Albert. 1998. *The Birth of Bioethics.* New York: Oxford University Press.

Jonsen, Albert, and Stephen Toulmin. 1988. *The Abuse of Casuistry: A History of Moral Reasoning.* Berkley, CA: University of California Press.

Juengst, Eric T. 1996. "Self-Critical Federal Science? The Ethics Experiment within the U.S. Human Genome Project." *Social Philosophy and Policy* 13, no. 2: 63–95.

Kant, Immanuel. [1785] 2005. *Fundamental Principles of the Metaphysics of Morals.* Translated by Thomas Kingsmill Abbot. Mineola, NY: Dover.

Kass Council (President's Council on Bioethics). 2002–2009. Minutes of public meetings available at http://www.bioethics.gov/.

———. 2002. *Human Cloning and Human Dignity: An Ethical Inquiry.* Washington, DC: U.S. Government Printing Office.

———. 2003a. *Beyond Therapy: Biotechnology and the Pursuit of Happiness.* Washington, DC: U.S. Government Printing Office. Another 2003 edition, New York: Harper Collins.

———. 2003b. *Being Human: Readings from the President's Council on Bioethics.* Washington, DC: U.S. Government Printing Office. 2004 edition, New York: W.W. Norton.

———. 2004a. *Monitoring Stem Cell Research.* Washington, DC: U.S. Government Printing Office.

———. 2004b. *Reproduction and Responsibility: The Regulation of New Biotechnologies.* Washington, DC: U.S. Government Printing Office.

———. 2005a. *White Paper: Alternative Sources of Pluripotent Stem Cells.* Washington, DC: U.S. Government Printing Office.

———. 2005b. *Taking Care: Ethical Caregiving in Our Aging Society.* Washington, DC: U.S. Government Printing Office.

———. 2008. *Human Dignity and Bioethics.* Washington, DC: U.S. Government Printing Office.

Kass, Leon. 1971. "The New Biology: What Price Relieving Man's Estate?" *Science* 174: 779–90.

———. 1979. "'Making Babies' Revisited." *Public Interest,* no. 54: 32–60.

———. 1985. *Toward a More Natural Science: Biology and Human Affairs.* New York: Free Press.

———. 1991. "Death with Dignity and the Sanctity of Life." In *A Time to Be Born and a Time to Die,* edited by B. S. Kogan, 117–45. New York: Aldine De Gruyter.

———. 1996. "The Troubled Dream of Nature as a Moral Guide." *Hastings Center Report,* 26, no. 6: 22–24.

———. 1997. "The End of Courtship." *Public Interest,* no. 126 (Winter): 39–63.

———. 2002. *Life, Liberty and the Defense of Dignity.* San Francisco: Encounter Books.

———. 2003. *The Beginning of Wisdom: Reading Genesis.* New York: Free Press.

———. 2004. "We Don't Play Politics with Science." *Washington Post,* March 3.

———. 2005. "Reflections on Public Bioethics: A View from the Trenches." *Kennedy Institute of Ethics Journal* 15, no. 3: 221–50.

Kass, Leon, and James Wilson. 1998. *The Ethics of Human Cloning.* Washington, DC: AEI Press.

Kelly, Henry, Ivan Oelrich, Steven Aftergood, and Benn H. Tannenbaum. 2004. "Flying Blind: The Rise, Fall, and Possible Resurrection of Science Policy Advice in the United States." Report by the Federation of American Scientists. N.p.: Federation of American Scientists.

Kelly, Susan. 2003. "Public Bioethics and Publics: Consensus, Boundaries, and Participation in Biomedical Science Policy." *Science, Technology, and Human Values* 28, no. 3: 339–64.

Kennedy, Donald. 2004. "Just Treat, or Enhance?" *Science* 304, no. 5667: 17.

Kinnell, Galway. 1980. "After Making Love We Hear Footsteps." In *Mortal Acts, Mortal Words.* Boston: Houghton Mifflin.

Kintisch, Eli. 2005. "Anticloning Forces Launch Second-Term Offensive." *Science* 307, no. 5716: 1702–3.

Kitcher, Philip. 2001. *Science, Truth, and Democracy.* New York: Oxford University Press.

Kleinman, Daniel Lee. 1995. *Politics on the Endless Frontier: Postwar Research Policy in the United States.* Durham, NC: Duke University Press.

Knaus, William, and Joanne Lynn. 2001. *Study to Understand Prognoses and Preferences for Outcomes and Risks of Treatment SUPPORT.* Ann Arbor, MI: Interuniversity Consortium for Political and Social Research.

Kohn, David, and Julie Bell. 2004. "2 Appointees Defend Place on Bioethics Panel: Bush Critics Say Politics, Not Science, Ruled Choice." *Baltimoresun.com,* March 2. http://www.baltimoresun.com/.

Korsgaard, Christine. 1996. *Sources of Normativity.* Cambridge: Cambridge University Press.

Kuehn, Thomas, and Alan Porter, eds. 1981. *Science, Technology, and National Policy.* Ithaca, NY: Cornell University Press.

Kuhn, Thomas. 1963. *The Structure of Scientific Revolutions.* Chicago: University of Chicago Press.

Kuklick, Bruce. 1977. *The Rise of American Philosophy: Cambridge, Massachusetts 1860–1930.* New Haven: Yale University Press.

Kymlicka, Will. 1989. *Liberalism, Community, and Culture.* Oxford: Oxford University Press.

Landau, Ralph, and Nathan Rosenberg, eds. 1986. *Positive Sum Strategy: Harnessing Technology for Economic Growth.* Washington, DC: National Academy Press.

Lane, Robert. 2000. *The Loss of Happiness in Market Democracies.* New Haven, CT: Yale University Press.

Larmore, Charles. 1987. *Patterns of Moral Complexity.* Cambridge: Cambridge University Press.

Lawler, Peter. 2002. *Aliens in America: The Strange Truth about Our Souls.* Wilmington, DE: ISI Books.

Leopold, Aldo. 1949. *A Sand County Almanac.* New York: Oxford University Press.

Levin, Yuval. 2000. *Tyranny of Reason: The Origins and Consequences of the Social Scientific Outlook.* Lanham, MD: University Press of America.

———. 2003. "The Paradox of Conservative Bioethics." *New Atlantis,* no. 1 (Spring): 53–65.

Lewis, C. S. 1965. *Perelandra: A Novel.* New York: Macmillan.

Lilla, Mark. 2007. *The Stillborn God: Religion, Politics, and the Modern West.* New York: Knopf.

Lindblom, Charles E. 1959. "The Science of 'Muddling Through.'" *Public Administration Review* 19: 79–88.

Lippmann, Walter. 1955. *The Public Philosophy.* New York: New American Library.

Lucena, Juan. 2005. *Defending the Nation: U.S. Policymaking to Create Scientists and Engineers from Sputnik to the "War against Terrorism."* Lanham, MD: University Press of America.

Lustig, Andrew. 2005. "After Kass: The Future of the President's Council on Bioethics." *Commonweal,* December 2: 7–8.

Machiavelli, Niccolò. [1532] 1976. *The Prince.* Translated by James B. Atkinson. Indianapolis, IN: Bobbs-Merrill.

MacIntyre, Alasdair. 1984. *After Virtue: A Study in Moral Theory.* Rev. 2nd ed. Notre Dame, IN: University of Notre Dame Press. (Orig. pub. 1981.)

———. 1988. *Whose Justice? Which Rationality?* Notre Dame, IN: University of Notre Dame Press.

Macklin, Ruth. 2006. "The New Conservatives in Bioethics: Who Are They and What Do They Seek?" *Hastings Center Report* 36, no. 1: 34–43.

Maclean, Anne. 1993. *The Elimination of Morality: Reflections on Utilitarianism and Bioethics.* New York: Routledge.

Macpherson, C. B. 1962. *The Political Theory of Possessive Individualism: Hobbes to Locke.* New York: Oxford University Press.

Majunder, Mary Anderlik. 2005. "Respecting Difference and Moving beyond Regulation: Tasks for U.S. Bioethics Commissions in the Twenty-First Century." *Kennedy Institute of Ethics Journal* 15, no. 3: 289–303.

Mappes, Thomas A., and David DeGrazia, eds. 2001. *Biomedical Ethics.* 5th ed. Boston: McGraw-Hill.

Mathieu, Deborah. 1994. "Another Forum for Bioethics in U.S. Public Policy?" *Politics and the Life Sciences* 13: 91–92.

May, William. 2005. "The President's Council on Bioethics: My Take on Some of its Deliberations." *Perspectives in Biology and Medicine* 48, no. 2: 229–40.

———. 2008. *Catholic Bioethics and the Gift of Human Life.* Huntington, IN: Our Sunday Visitor.

McClay, Wilfred. 2004. "Science and Self-Government." *New Atlantis,* no. 4 (Winter): 17–22.

McGinn, Robert. 1991. *Science, Technology, and Society.* Upper Saddle River, NJ: Prentice Hall.

McKibben, Bill. 2003. *Enough: Staying Human in an Engineered Age.* New York: Times Books.

Meilaender, Gilbert. 1995. *Body, Soul, and Bioethics.* Notre Dame, IN: University of Notre Dame Press.

Merleau-Ponty, Maurice. 1962. *The Phenomenology of Perception.* London: Routledge and Kegan Paul.

Merton, Thomas. 1964. *Seeds of Destruction.* New York: Farrar, Straus and Giroux.

Meslin, Eric. 2004. "The President's Council on Bioethics: Fair and Balanced?" *Hastings Center Report* 32, no. 2: 6–8.

Michaels, David, et al. 2002. "Advice without Dissent." *Science* 298, no. 5594: 703.

Midgley, Mary. 1978. *Beast and Man: The Roots of Human Nature.* London: Routledge.

Mill, John Stuart. 1963–1991. *Collected Works of John Stuart Mill.* 33 vols. Edited by J. M. Robson. Toronto: University of Toronto Press.

Miller, Stephen. 2007. *Conversation: A History of a Declining Art.* New Haven, CT: Yale University Press.

Mooney, Chris. 2001. "Irrationalist in Chief." *American Prospect* 12, no. 17 (Sept. 24–Oct. 8).

———. 2005. *The Republican War on Science.* New York: Basic Books.

Moreno, Jonathan. 1995. *Deciding Together: Bioethics and Moral Consensus.* New York: Oxford University Press.

———. 1999. *Undue Risk: Secret State Experiments on Humans.* New York: W. H. Freeman.

———. 2005. "The End of the Great Bioethics Compromise." *Hastings Center Report* 35, no. 1: 14–15.

Mulhall, Stephen, and Adam Swift. 1992. *Liberals and Communitarians.* Oxford: Blackwell.

Murdoch, Iris. 1971. *The Sovereignty of Good.* London: Routledge.

Murray, Iain. 2005. "Bioethics Panel Illustrates Scientific Ethics' Complexity." *Tech Central Station* (March 14).

Myers, David. 2000. *The American Paradox: Spiritual Hunger in an Age of Plenty.* New Haven, CT: Yale University Press.

NAS (National Academies Committee on Science, Engineering, and Public Policy). 2002. *Scientific and Medical Aspects of Human Reproductive Cloning.* Washington, DC: National Academies Press. See National Academies Committee on Science, Engineering, and Public Policy.

———. 2004. *Science and Technology in the National Interest: Ensuring the Best Presidential and Federal Advisory Committee Science and Technology Appointments.* Washington, DC: National Academies Press.

———. 2005. *Rising Above the Gathering Storm: Energizing and Employing America for a Brighter Economic Future.* Washington, DC: National Academies Press.

National Academies Committee on Science, Engineering, and Public Policy. See NAS.

NBAC (National Bioethics Advisory Commission). 1997. *Cloning Human Beings.* Bethesda, MD: U.S. Government Printing Office.

———. 1999. *Ethical Issues in Human Stem Cell Research.* Bethesda, MD: U.S. Government Printing Office.

———. 2001. *Ethical and Policy Issues in Research Involving Human Participants.* Bethesda, MD: U.S. Government Printing Office.

National Bioethics Advisory Committee. See NBAC.

National Commission for the Protection of Human Subjects of Biomedical and Behavioral Research. 1979. *The Belmont Report: Ethical Principles and Guidelines for the Protection of Human Subjects of Research.* Washington, DC: U.S. Government Printing Office.

Nature Biotechnology. 2003. "Beyond Belief." *Nature Biotechnology* 21: 1411.

Nietzsche, Friedrich. 1954. *The Portable Nietzsche*. Translated by Walter Kaufmann. New York: Viking Press.

———. 1967. *The Will to Power*. Translated by Walter Kaufmann. New York: Vintage.

———. 1974. *Basic Writings of Nietzsche*. Translated by Walter Kaufmann. New York: Vintage.

Nelson, James. 2005. "The Baroness's Committee and the President's Council: Ambition and Alienation in Public Bioethics." *Kennedy Institute of Ethics Journal* 15, no. 3: 251–67.

Nelson, W. R., ed. 1968. *The Politics of Science*. New York: Oxford University Press.

Noah, Timothy. 2004. "Leon Kass, You Silly Ass! Please Stop Denying You Tilted the Bioethics Panel." *MSN Slate Magazine*, March 8. http://www.slate.com/.

Norton, Anne. 2004. *Leo Strauss and the Politics of American Empire*. New Haven: Yale University Press.

Nozick, Robert. 1974. *Anarchy, State, and Utopia*. New York: Basic Books.

Nussbaum, Martha. 2004. *Hiding from Humanity: Disgust, Shame, and the Law*. Princeton, NJ: Princeton University Press.

Oakeshott, Michael. 1989. *The Voice of Liberal Learning: Michael Oakeshott on Education*. Edited by Timothy Fuller. New Haven, CT: Yale University Press.

Olson, Richard. 2008. *Science and Scientism in Nineteenth-Century Europe*. Champaign, IL: University of Illinois Press.

Pellegrino, Edmund. 1999. "The Origins and Evolution of Bioethics: Some Personal Reflections." *Kennedy Institute of Ethics Journal* 9, no. 1: 73–88.

Pielke, Roger, Jr. 2005. "Defending Kass But Confirming the Conflict." Center for Science and Technology Policy Research, March 18. http://sciencepolicy.colorado.edu/prometheus/archives/biotechnology/000379defending_kass_but_c.html.

———. 2007. *The Honest Broker: Making Sense of Science in Policy and Politics*. Cambridge: Cambridge University Press.

Pielke, Roger Jr., ed. 2004. "A Report on the Misuse of Science in the Administrations of George H. W. Bush and William J. Clinton." http://sciencepolicy.colorado.edu/admin/publication_files/resource-1935-2004.27.pdf.

Pielke, Roger, Jr., and Radford Byerly, Jr. 1998. "Beyond Basic and Applied." *Physics Today* 51, no. 2: 42–46.

Pinker, Steven. 2008. "The Stupidity of Dignity: Conservative Bioethics' Latest Most Dangerous Ploy." *New Republic*, May 28.

Plato. 1961. *Collected Dialogues of Plato*. Edited by Edith Hamilton and Huntington Cairns. Princeton, NJ: Princeton University Press.

Poland, Susan Cartier. 1998. "Bioethics Commissions: Town Meetings with a 'Blue, Blue Ribbon.'" *Kennedy Institute of Ethics Journal* 8, no. 1: 91–109.

Potter, Van Renesselar. 1971. *Bioethics: Bridge to the Future*. Englewood Cliffs, NJ: Prentice-Hall.

President's Commission for the Study of Ethical Problems in Medicine and Biomedical and Behavioral Research. 1981. *Defining Death: Medical, Legal, and Ethical Issues in the Determination of Death.* Washington, DC: U.S. Government Printing Office.

———. 1982. *Making Health Care Decisions: The Ethical and Legal Implications of Informed Consent in the Patient-Practitioner Relationship.* Washington, DC: U.S. Government Printing Office.

———. 1983. *Deciding to Forgo Life-Sustaining Treatment: Ethical, Medical, and Legal Issues in Treatment Decisions.* Washington, DC: U.S. Government Printing Office.

———. 1983. *Securing Access to Health Care: The Ethical Implications of Differences in the Availability of Health Services.* Washington, DC: U.S. Government Printing Office.

President's Council on Bioethics. See Kass Council.

Price, Don K. 1965. *The Scientific Estate.* Cambridge, MA: Belknap Press.

Primack, Joel, and Frank von Hippel. 1974. *Advice and Dissent: Scientists in the Political Arena.* New York: Basic Books.

Putnam, Hilary. 2002. *The Collapse of the Fact/Value Dichotomy and Other Essays.* Cambridge, MA: Harvard University Press.

Ramsey, Paul. 1970. *Fabricated Man: The Ethics of Genetic Control.* New Haven: Yale University Press.

———. 1976. "Prolonged Dying: Not Medically Indicated." *Hastings Center Report* 6, no. 1: 14–17.

Rawls, John. 1971. *A Theory of Justice.* Cambridge, MA: Harvard University Press.

———. 1975. "A Kantian Conception of Equality." *Cambridge Review* 96, no. 2225 (Feb.): 94–99.

———. 1980. "Kantian Constructivism in Moral Theory." *Journal of Philosophy* 77: 515–72.

———. 1993. *Political Liberalism.* New York: Columbia University Press.

Raz, Joseph. 1986. *The Morality of Freedom.* Oxford: Oxford University Press.

Roco, Mihail, and William Bainbridge. 2002. *Converging Technologies for Improving Human Performance.* A Report Funded by the National Science Foundation. New York: Springer.

Rorty, Richard. 1979. *Philosophy and the Mirror of Nature.* Princeton, NJ: Princeton University Press.

Rosen, Christine. 2004. "Good Council: A Review of Two Recent Reports from the President's Council on Bioethics." Ethics and Public Policy Center, July 13. http://www.eppc.org/publications/pubID.2141/pub_detail.asp.

Rosenberg, Charles. 1999. "Meanings, Policies, and Medicine: On the Bioethical Enterprise and History." *Daedalus* 128, no. 4: 27–46.

Rousseau, Jean-Jacques. [1754] 1994. *Discourse on the Origin and Foundations of Inequality.* Translated by Philip Franklin. Oxford: Oxford University Press.

Rothman, David J. 2004. "Research, Human: Historical Aspects." In *Encyclopedia of Bioethics*, 3rd ed., edited by Stephen Post, 2316–26. New York: Macmillan.

Sabatier, Paul, ed. 1999. *Theories of the Policy Process*. Boulder, CO: Westview Press.

Sacks, Jonathan. 2003. *The Dignity of Difference: How to Avoid the Clash of Civilizations*. London: Continuum.

Saletan, William. 2002. "Bush's Mutant Cloning Report." *MSN Slate Magazine*, July 6. http://www.slate.com/.

———. 2004. "Govern This." *MSN Slate Magazine*, December 4. http://www.slate.com/.

———. 2005. "Who's Right in the Bioethics Debates." *MSN Slate Magazine*, October 14. http://www.slate.com/.

Sandel, Michael. 1982. *Liberalism and the Limits of Justice*. London: Cambridge University Press.

———. 1996. "America's Search for a New Public Philosophy." *Atlantic Monthly* 277, no. 3 (March): 57–74.

———. 2004. "The Case against Perfection." *Atlantic Monthly* 293, no. 3 (April): 51–62.

———. 2007. *The Case against Perfection: Ethics in the Age of Genetic Engineering*. Cambridge, MA: Belknap Press.

Sarewitz, Daniel. 1996. *Frontiers of Illusion: Science, Technology, and the Politics of Progress*. Philadelphia: Temple University Press.

———. 1997. "Science and Environmental Policy: An Excess of Objectivity." In *Earth Matters: The Earth Sciences, Philosophy, and the Claims of Community*, edited by Robert Frodeman, 79–98. Upper Saddle River, NJ: Prentice Hall.

———. 2004. "How Science Makes Environmental Controversies Worse," *Environmental Science and Policy* 7, no. 5: 385–403.

Sartre, Jean-Paul. 1958. *Existentialism and Humanism*. Translated by Philip Mairet. London: Methuen.

Scanlon, T.M. 1998. *What We Owe to Each Other*. Cambridge, MA: Belknap Press.

Schattschneider, E.E. 1960. *The Semisovereign People: A Realist's View of Democracy in America*. New York: Holt, Rinehart, and Winston.

Schaub, Diana. 2003. "Slavery Plus Abortion." *Public Interest*, no. 150 (Winter): 41–46.

Schneewind, Jerome B. 1998. *The Invention of Autonomy: A History of Modern Moral Philosophy*. Cambridge: Cambridge University Press.

Sclove, Richard E. 1995. *Democracy and Technology*. New York: Guilford Press

Shalit, Ruth. 1997. "When We Were Philosopher Kings." *New Republic*, April 28.

Shapley, Deborah, and Rustum Roy. 1985. *Lost at the Frontier: U.S. Science and Technology Policy Adrift*. Philadelphia: ISI Press.

Sher, George. 1997. *Beyond Neutrality: Perfectionism and Politics*. Cambridge: Cambridge University Press.

Shorto, Russell. 2006. "Contra-Contraception." *New York Times Magazine*, May 7.

Singer, Peter. 1972. "Moral Experts." *Analysis* 32: 115–17.

Smith, Bruce. 1990. *American Science Policy since World War II*. Washington, DC: Brookings Institution.

Smith, Wesley. 2003. "Kass, in the Firing Line." *National Review Online*, December 5. http://www.nationalreview.com.

Snow, C. P. 1959. *The Two Cultures and the Scientific Revolution*. Cambridge: Cambridge University Press.

Sonnert, Gerhard, and Gerald Holton. 2002. *Ivory Bridges: Connecting Science and Society*. Cambridge, MA: MIT Press.

Soper, Kate. 1995. *What Is Nature? Culture, Politics, and the Non-human*. Malden, MA: Wiley-Blackwell.

Stevens, M. L. Tina. 2000. *Bioethics in America: Origins and Cultural Politics*. Baltimore, MD: Johns Hopkins University Press.

Stokes, Donald. 1997. *Pasteur's Quadrant: Basic Science and Technological Innovation*. Washington, DC: Brookings Institution.

Strauss, Leo. 1953. *Natural Right and History*. Chicago: University of Chicago Press.

———. [1968] 1989. *Liberalism Ancient and Modern*. Chicago: University of Chicago Press.

Struhkamp, Rita M. 2005. "Patient Autonomy: A View from the Kitchen." *Medicine, Healthcare, and Philosophy* 8: 105–14.

Suchman, Mark. C. 1995. "Managing Legitimacy: Strategic and Institutional Approaches." *Academy of Management Review* 20, no. 3: 571–610.

Sunstein, Cass. 2007. *Republic.com 2.0*. Princeton, NJ: Princeton University Press.

Taylor, Charles. 1989. *Sources of the Self: The Making of the Modern Identity*. Cambridge, MA: Harvard University Press.

———. 1991. *The Ethics of Authenticity*. Cambridge, MA: Harvard University Press.

Taylor, Gordon. 1968. *Biological Time Bomb*. New York: World Publishers.

Toffler, Alvin. 1970. *Future Shock*. New York: Random House.

Toulmin, Stephen. 1982. "How Medicine Saved the Life of Ethics." *Perspectives in Biology and Medicine* 2, no. 4: 736–50.

———. 2001. *Return to Reason*. Cambridge, MA: Harvard University Press.

Tronto, J. C. 1993. *Moral Boundaries: A Political Argument for an Ethic of Care*. New York: Routledge.

Turner, Leigh. 2003. "Has the President's Council on Bioethics Missed the Boat?" *British Medical Journal* 327: 629.

———. 2004. "Science, Politics, and the President's Council on Bioethics." *Nature Biotechnology* 22: 509–10.

UNESCO (United Nations Educational, Scientific, and Cultural Organization Division of Ethics of Science and Technology). 2005. *Bioethics Committees at Work: Procedures and Policies*. Paris: UNESCO.

Union of Concerned Scientists. 2004. *Scientific Integrity in Policymaking: An Investigation into the Bush Administration's Misuse of Science.* http://www.ucsusa.org/.

United Nations Educational, Scientific, and Cultural Organization Division of Ethics of Science and Technology. See UNESCO.

United States General Accounting Office. See USGAO.

United States Office of Technology Assessment. See USOTA.

USGAO. 2004. *Federal Advisory Committees: Additional Guidance Could Help Agencies Better Ensure Independence and Balance.* GAO-04-328. Washington, DC: U.S. Government Printing Office.

USOTA (United States Office of Technology Assessment). 1993. *Biomedical Ethics in U.S. Public Policy.* OTA-PB-BBS-105. Washington, DC: U.S. Government Printing Office.

Van Der Burg, Wibren, and Theo van Willigenburg, eds. 1998. *Reflective Equilibrium: Essays in Honor of Robert Heeger.* London: Springer.

Veatch, Robert M. 2003. *Basics of Bioethics.* 2nd ed. Upper Saddle River, NJ: Prentice Hall.

Vogel, Lawrence. 2006. "Natural-Law Judaism? The Genesis of Bioethics in Hans Jonas, Leo Strauss, and Leon Kass." *Hastings Center Report* (May–June): 32–44.

Wade, Nicholas. 2009. "Obama Plans to Replace Bush's Bioethics Panel," *New York Times,* June 17.

Wall, Steven, and George Klosko. 2003. *Perfectionism and Neutrality: Essays in Liberal Theory.* Lanham, MD: Rowman & Littlefield.

Walzer, Michael. 1981. "Philosophy and Democracy." *Political Theory* 9: 379–400.

Waxman, Henry A. 2003. *Politics and Science in the Bush Administration.* Report Prepared by the U.S. House of Representatives Committee on Government Reform, Minority Staff. http://oversighthouse.gov/.

Weiss, Rick. 2002. "Bush Unveils Bioethics Council." *Washington Post,* January 17.

———. 2005. "Conservatives Draft a 'Bioethics Agenda' for President." *Washington Post,* March 7.

Wildavsky, Aaron. 1964. *The Politics of the Budgetary Process.* Boston: Little, Brown.

Wilkie, Dana. 2002. "The Puzzle of Leon Kass." *Crisis* (May/June). Available at http://lynnkramer.tblog.com/post/303756.

Wilson, James Q. 2005. "On Leon Kass and Bioethics." *TCS Daily,* March 17. http://tcsdaily.com/Article.aspx?id=031705G.

Winner, Langdon. 2004. "Technologies as Forms of Life." In *Readings in the Philosophy of Technology,* edited by David Kaplan, 103–14. Lanham, MD: Rowman and Littlefield.

Wolanin, Thomas. 1975. *Presidential Advisory Commissions: Truman to Nixon.* Madison, WI: University of Wisconsin Press.

Wolbring, Gregor. 2008. "Is There an End to Out-able? Is There an End to the Rat Race for Abilities?" *Media and Culture* 11, no. 3. http://journal.media-culture .org.au/index.php/mcjournal/article/viewArticle/57.

Wolfson, Adam. 2000. *The Liberal Tradition in Focus: Problems and New Perspectives.* Lanham, MD: Lexington Books.

———. 2003. "Why Conservatives Care About Biotechnology." *New Atlantis,* no. 2 (Summer): 55–64.

Wright, Robert. 2001. "Fearful New World." *MSN Slate Magazine,* August 11. http:// www.slate.com/.

Yoder, Scot. 1998. "The Nature of Ethical Expertise." *Hastings Center Report* 28, no. 6: 11–19.

INDEX

Abu Ghraib, 181n.9
advance directives, 82–84
advisory committees. *See* federal
  advisory committees
aging, 81–85
alethia, 164
American Society for Cell Biology, 139
Aristotle
  compared to Mill, 53
  on cultivation and construction, 99
  on happiness, 107
  on humans as rational animals, 87
  implications for bioethics, 42–46,
    184nn.2–4
  on philosopher's method, 178–79
  and teleology, 95
  on virtue, 186n.3
Arnhart, Larry, 96
autonomy. *See also* Kant, Immanuel
  and advance directives, 82–84
  and aging, 81, 84
  and enhancement, 105
  and human nature, 171
  and liberal education, 73
  and nested goods, 91
  origins of concept, 180n.1
  and respect for persons, 23–24

Baby Doe regulations, 181n.6
Bacon, Francis, 48, 49, 97
Belmont Report, 22, 23, 24, 29, 151,
  161, 169
Berkowitz, Peter, 121

Berlin, Isaiah, 168, 171, 177
Beyond Therapy, 101–12
Big Science, 153
Bildung, 177
bioconservative, 116, 117
bioethics
  ancient roots of, 41–47
  "nature" used in bioethical
    discourse, 97–101
  origins of term, 42, 181n.10, 184n.1
bioethics committees. *See* public
  bioethics commissions
Biomedical Ethics Advisory
  Committee (BEAC), 26
bios, 45, 89
biotechnology, 2, 8, 37, 44, 106, 108
Blackburn, Elizabeth, 120, 126,
  139–40, 141–44
Blackford, Russell, 98
Bonds, Barry, 102–3
Borgmann, Albert, 68–69
Bostrom, Nick, 100
Brave New World, 107, 110
Brink, David, 178
Brooks, Harvey, 157
Brownback, Sam, 145
Bush, George W., 1, 30, 31, 32, 122,
  139, 180n.1
Bush, Vannevar, 156, 158, 193n.13

Callahan, Daniel, 31, 184n.1
capitalism, 54
Caplan, Arthur, 125, 190n.10

Carson, Benjamin, 140
Carson, Rachel, 162
Charo, R. Alta, 121, 125
child labor, 162
cloning. *See Human Cloning and
Human Dignity*; instrumentalism,
and cloning; National Bioethics
Advisory Commission, on cloning; rich bioethics, on cloning;
somatic cell nuclear transfer
co-creator. *See* playing God
Cohen, Eric, 121
Comte, Auguste, 185n.14
conflict of interest, 145–46
contraception, 99
contract. *See* social contract
conversation, 174–79
culture, 90–91, 97–99, 161–62
culture wars, 124

Dahl, Robert, 168
Darwin, Charles, 51, 88, 96
democratic legitimacy, 132–37, 140,
144, 146, 147–48, 170, 191n.5
depression, 109
Descartes, René, 49–51, 87
de Tocqueville, Alexis, 161
Dewey, John, 154
Diamond, Cora, 163–65
Dickey Amendment, 31
Dickson, David, 193n.7
dignity, 88, 103–4, 106, 161
Dresser, Rebecca, 127
drugs, 108

Elliott, Carl, 70–71, 86, 126, 129
embryonic stem cells. *See* stem cell
research
Engelhardt, Tristram, Jr., 57–59
enhancement, 65–67, 70–71,
100–101. *See also* rich bioethics,
on enhancement

Ethical, Legal, and Social Impacts
(ELSI) program, 27, 150
Ethics Advisory Board (EAB), 24–25
ethics advisory bodies, 134–35, 138,
151
eugenics, 65–66, 99–100
Evans, John, 33, 76, 169–70, 172
experts
and bioethics commissions, 18–19,
22, 29–30, 35–36
and democracy, 131–35, 168–70
as honest brokers or issue
advocates, 137–38
and Kass Council membership, 119
and policy, 152–54
and Stoics as *technè*, 44

fact-value divide, 90, 93–95, 99
Federal Advisory Committee Act
(FACA), 135, 190n.6
federal advisory committees, 125,
135, 169
Federation of American Scientists, 125
Feenberg, Andrew, 162
final causes. *See* teleology
Fish, Stanley, 165
Fletcher, Joseph, 47
Foster, Daniel, 120
Foucault, Michel, 188n.12
friendship, 175
Fukuyama, Francis, 120, 129, 188n.6

Gazzaniga, Michael, 120, 127, 129,
140, 192n.9
General Accounting Office (GAO),
125, 136
George, Robert, 119, 126, 173, 190n.11
Glendon, Mary Ann, 119, 130
gnosticism, 47–48
Gómez-Lobo, Alfonso, 119, 129, 130
great divide, 41
Greenberg, Daniel, 157

Haldane, J. B. S., 153
happiness, 107–11, 158
Haraway, Donna, 90
harm, 74, 78
harm principle, 56
Hawthorne, Nathaniel, 149
health care, 158
Heidegger, Martin, 64, 162, 164,
    185n.12
Heisenberg, Werner, 153
Herder, Johann, 168
higher-order volitions, 91
Hippocrates, 43
Hobbes, Thomas, 39, 53, 55, 61, 152,
    168, 185n.13
honest broker, 137–38, 145
Human Cloning and Human Dignity,
    76–80
human dignity. *See* dignity
human experimentation. *See* research
    with human subjects
human nature, 89–93, 95, 97–100,
    102, 152, 171
human rights, 93
Hume, David, 93, 188n.7–8

identity, 61–62, 79, 108–11
informed consent, 14, 24, 25, 30, 62, 84
informed desire satisfaction, 177–78
innovation, 155–58
institutional review boards (IRBs), 18
instrumentalism
    and aging and caregiving, 81–85
    and cloning, 76
    defined, 4–6
    and enhancement, 103–11
    as formal rationality, 6, 33–36
    and happiness, 107
    as insufficient frame for bioethical
        inquiry, 63, 86, 112, 117
    as isolationist, 6, 85
    as lacking diversity, 119

and mind-body dualism, 88–89
and neutrality, 71, 121
and policy, 150–51, 157, 159
as presupposing a value-neutral
    view of technology, 64
as recapitulating modern
    liberalism, 57–60, 62
as technocracy, 170
in vitro fertilization (IVF), 25, 31, 80
iron triangle, 154

Jonas, Hans, 52, 96–97, 189n.15

Kant, Immanuel
    autonomy, 13, 15, 39, 52–53,
        185n.16
    "Dare to know," 13
    and human nature, 88–90
Kass, Leon
    accused by Blackburn and Rowley,
        143–44
    accused of conflict of interest,
        145–46
    appointed to council by President
        Bush, 32
    on Bible, 45
    on Blackburn's dismissal, 139–40
    on Carson, 140
    intellectual biography, 117–19
    on liberal education, 173
    meeting with President Bush, 31–32
    on mission of the council, 3, 33,
        36–37, 144
    on norms guiding the council, 136,
        191n.13
    on process of selecting topics, 123
    skepticism about science and
        technology, 32
Kennedy, John F., 186n.19
Kepler, Johannes, 49
Kinnell, Galway, 165
Kitcher, Philip, 170

Lawler, Peter, 119
legitimacy. *See* democratic legitimacy
Leopold, Aldo, 162
Levin, Yuval, 121
Lewis, C. S., 45
liberal education, 73, 173–74, 177
liberalism
    foundations of, 55–56
    and human nature, 92–93
    implications for bioethics, 56–60
    neutrality of, 62, 68–75
    and pluralism, 171–73
    and scientific expertise, 152–53
life, 45, 52
lifeworld, 88–89
linear model, 156
Lippmann, Walter, 86, 174
living will. *See* advance directives
Locke, John, 53, 54, 61, 168

Machiavelli, Niccolò, 48, 55, 152
MacIntyre, Alisdair, 42, 93
Macpherson, C. B., 56
Maimonides, Moses, 181n.4
Marx, Karl, 54
Maslow's hierarchy of needs, 91
May, William, 119
McHugh, Paul, 119
medical ethics, 194n.1
medicalization, 111
Meilander, Gilbert, 119, 129
memory, 108–9
Merleau-Ponty, Maurice, 88
Merton, Thomas, 166
Midgley, Mary, 90, 94, 188nn.9, 11
Mill, John Stuart, 53, 54, 56, 75, 92, 108, 177
mind-body dualism, 87–90
misuse of science, 141–43
modernity, 48–49, 68
modern science, 49
monism, 168, 171

mood, 108–11
moral friends and strangers, 57–58
Moreno, Jonathan, 129, 182n.24
Muir, John, 162
Murdoch, Iris, 39

National Academy of Science (NAS), 28, 125
National Bioethics Advisory Commission (NBAC)
    on cloning, 76–80
    formation of, 29–30
    traveling, 122
National Commission for the Protection of Human Subjects of Biomedical and Behavioral Research (National Commission), 21–22
National Institutes of Health (NIH), 18, 21, 22, 27, 31, 32, 118
National Neural Technology Initiative, 67
National Science Foundation (NSF), 66
naturalistic fallacy, 93, 97. *See also* fact-value divide
natural law, 44
Newton, Isaac, 51
Nietzsche, Friedrich, 53, 54, 177
Nozick, Robert, 107–9
Nuremberg Code, 14, 57, 181n.3
Nussbaum, Martha, 88

Oakeshott, Michael, 174
Obama, Barack, 8
Office of Technology Assessment, 27
open instincts, 90

Pellegrino, Edmund, 180n.1
Pellegrino Council, 161, 180n.1, 194n.5
perfectionism, 72, 73, 172–73
personal identity. *See* identity
Pielke, Roger, 137, 154

Pinker, Stephen, 194n.5
Plato, 42–46, 168, 172, 175, 184n.2
playing God, 44–45, 47
pluralism, 57–59, 168, 171, 176,
    178–79
politicization, 136–37
politicization of science, 125–26
positive liberty, 177
postnormal science, 155
Potter, Van Renesselar, 184n.1
President's Commission for the
    Study of Ethical Problems in
    Medicine and Biomedical
    and Behavioral Research
    (President's Commission), 25
principlism, 22–24, 182n.18
proxy directives, 85
Prozac, 109
public bioethics commissions
    academic debate pertaining to
        merits of, 26–29
    congressional debate pertaining to
        formation of, 19–21
    definition of, 22, 182n.15
    functions or goals of, 18–19, 26,
        34–37, 180n.3, 192n.2
    within humanities policy, 159
    and liberal democracy, 72–75, 168,
        173
    outside the U.S., 27, 183n.33
public philosophy, 171–73

Ramsey, Paul, 47, 119
Rawls, John, 69–70, 71, 74
Raz, Joseph, 73
Recombinant DNA Advisory
    Committee, 181n.11
renal dialysis, 15
reprogenetics, 80
research with human subjects
    by Nazis, 14
    significant cases, 16–17
responsible science movement, 181n.8

Riccardo, David, 54
rich bioethics
    on aging and caregiving, 81–85
    as antidote to instrumentalism or
        the thinning of public bioethical
        debate, 35, 60, 63–64, 68, 86,
        189n.19
    benefits of, 8
    on cloning, 76–80, 119, 136, 141,
        187n.9
    in contrast to previous bioethics
        committees, 3
    on enhancement, 101–12
    as framing contrary to modern
        myths, 41
    and informed desire satisfaction, 177
    as institution, 115–16
    as legitimate aspect of liberal
        government, 69–75, 169
    as liberal education, 73, 173–74
    as liberalism without hiding, 88
    and membership, 116–17
    as middle way between tyranny and
        nihilism, 59
    and mission, 122, 143–44
    and neutrality of effect and
        justification, 71–72
    as partisan politics, 37–38
    as perfectionism, 172–73
    as policy relevant, 80–81
    as politicized and irrelevant, 7, 116,
        124–30
    and procedures, 121–23
    as public forum, 36, 40–41
    science and technology creating the
        need for, 77
    as substantive and holistic, 6
Rousseau, Jean-Jacques, 53, 59, 92
Rowley, Janet, 120, 126, 140, 141–44,
    192n.9

Saint-Simon, Henri de, 152
Sandel, Michael, 120, 168, 194n.3

Sarewitz, Daniel, 159, 192n.3
Sartre, Jean-Paul, 90
Schaub, Diana, 129
Schiavo, Terri, 124
science
    advisory bodies, 134
    and aging, 81, 86
    and bioethics, 5–6, 16, 19–20, 35,
        40–41, 77, 88–89, 129
    and fact-value dichotomy, 94–95
    and Hobbes, 40
    and humanities, 160, 165
    implications for ethics, 53
    implications for liberal democracy,
        2, 5–6, 8, 53, 60, 134–37,
        170–74
    and Kass, 117–18, 140
    misuse, 141–43
    modern origins of, 48–52
    and policy instrumentalism, 150
    President Bush, remarks on, 32
    and Stoics, 44
    and teleology, 95–97, 132, 134,
        153–54
science policy, 3, 7, 19, 26, 123, 128,
    137, 151–58
science studies, 132–33
secularization, 186n.21
selective serotonin reuptake inhibitors
    (SSRIs), 109
sex, 98–99
smart pills, 67
Smith, Adam, 54
social contract, 61, 64, 158, 159,
    186n.2
social science, 159, 170, 193n.14
Socrates
    on friendship, 175
    implications for bioethics, 43, 46
    on philosopher kings, 167
    on the polis, 61
somatic cell nuclear transfer (SCNT),
    76

Soper, Kate, 98
species, 91
Spinoza, Benedict, 55
stealth advocate, 138
stem cell research, 1, 30, 31, 142–44
steroids, 103–5
Stevenson, Adlai, 156
Stoics, 44, 47
Stokes, Donald, 193n.9
Strauss, Leo, 44, 184n.2
subjectivism, 171–72, 178

Taylor, Frederick Winslow, 153
technocracy, 152, 170
technology
    and aging, 81–82
    and bioethics, 5–6, 19, 26, 47, 60,
        77, 88–89, 124
    and cloning, 76, 80
    and constructivism, 90
    and enhancement, 101–11
    as form of life, 64–65, 72
    implications for liberal democracy,
        2, 5–6, 8, 40–41, 60, 68–75,
        85–86, 168, 171–77
    and Kass, 117
    and modernity, 49–50, 59
    and policy instrumentalism,
        156–58, 166
    as value neutral, 54, 64–68
teleology, 42, 50, 95–97
therapy/enhancement distinction,
    101–2
Thoreau, Henry David, 162
Toulmin, Stephen, 194n.1
Tuskegee Syphilis Experiment, 17

Vico, Giambattista, 168
virtues, 54

Warnock, Mary, 129
Wilson, James, 146
Wolfson, Adam, 121

ADAM BRIGGLE

is assistant professor of philosophy at the University of North Texas.